The Author

Sara Meeks, P.T., G.C.S. is a physical therapist, in practice for 36 years, who specializes in the treatment of osteoporosis, postural problems, back pain, and problems of the frail elderly. She is an American Physical Therapy Association certified Geriatric Clinical Specialist and chairperson of the Special Interest Group on Osteoporosis of the Section on Geriatrics.

The author has developed an easy, unique program for the prevention and treatment of osteoporosis, which has been highly successful with her patients. For the past two years she has been training physical therapists, physical therapist assistants, massage therapists, and exercise specialists across the country how to apply her program to the treatment of their own patients, and has presented her work at the state and national level.

Sara is a marathon runner, masters national and world champion in olympic weight-lifting, and certified Kripalu yoga instructor. She also works with mature athletes (runners and weightlifters) on injury prevention. She lives with her husband, John Harrison, a massage therapist, champion weightlifter and olympic weightlifting coach, and her four black cats, in Gainesville, Florida.

WALK TALL!

An Exercise Program for the
Prevention and Treatment of Osteoporosis

Sara Meeks, P.T., G.C.S.

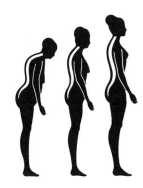

TRIAD PUBLISHING COMPANY   GAINESVILLE, FLORIDA

Printed in the United States of America

Library of Congress Cataloging-in-Publication Data

Meeks, Sara, 1940-
    Walk tall! : an exercise program for the prevention and treatment
of osteoporosis / Sara Meeks.
       p.   cm.
    Includes index.
    ISBN 0-937404-54-3 (pbk.)
      1. Posture disorders–Exercise therapy–popular works. 2. Backache–
Exercise therapy–Popular works. 3. Osteoporosis–Exercise therapy–
Popular works. 4. Osteopenia–Exercise therapy–Popular works. I. Title.
RD762.M44   1998
617.5' 6062–DC21   98-34433
                                              CIP

Published and distributed by Triad Publishing Company
Post Office Drawer 13355, Gainesville, FL 32604

To my aunt, Mary Helen Kelly, a woman who faced great physical challenges in her lifetime, who believed in me, and who always supported and encouraged me in my chosen field of physical therapy.

I would like to thank my husband, John Harrison, who is one of my most ardent supporters, who gives me encouragement when I falter, and without whom I would not be in a position to write this book.

I also would like to acknowledge all the people with osteoporosis with whom I have worked. Their courage and dedication have been inspirational.

CONTENTS

Preface, 9

Introduction, 11

I. Mental Imagery: "Yes, You Can Be Taller!" 13

II. Site-Specific Exercises, 15

III. Balance, 52

IV. Walking, 59

V. Scapular Stabilization, 63

VI. Activities of Daily Living, 69

VII. What's Next? 85

Glossary, 89

Index, 91

PREFACE

Osteoporosis crosses all ages, ethnic groups, genders, and lifestyles. Do not be too sure that you do not have or cannot get this life threatening condition.

OSTEOPOROSIS IS OCCURRING in epidemic proportions across this country and around the world. Many of you may believe you have no need to be concerned. But you really do. I have worked with people in all stages of this condition—young and old, male and female, of various ethnic origins, athletes and non-athletes—and I can tell you that it is truly EVERYONE'S problem.

I recently gave a seminar at which a 28-year-old, well-built, healthy looking man stood up and volunteered the information that he had recently been diagnosed with osteoporosis by bone density scan. To look at him, it was impossible to tell.

Do any of these statements apply to you?

"I am a man; therefore I cannot have osteoporosis."

"I am a teenager; therefore I cannot have osteoporosis."

"I am taking estrogen; therefore I cannot have osteoporosis."

"I take calcium, exercise regularly, don't smoke or drink; therefore I cannot have osteoporosis."

"There is no history of osteoporosis in my family; therefore I cannot have it."

"I do not have back pain; therefore I do not have osteoporosis."

If you agree with even one of these statements and you do not see osteoporosis as your problem, you need to open your eyes. Although some people are more at risk than others, this life threatening condition crosses all ages, ethnic groups, genders, and lifestyle considerations.

The good news is that osteoporosis can usually be prevented; if you already have it, it can be treated. But if you expect to live independently into old age, you must take action as early as possible.

Do you do sit-ups, abdominal crunches and leg lifts in an effort to strengthen the abdominal area? These forward-bending exercises compress the spine. And if you have low bone mass they will increase your risk of a compression fracture. Unfortunately, most people with low bone mass do not know it.

There is much information available on osteoporosis, but not all of it is correct. To reduce your risk of fracture you must become an informed consumer: ask questions, request a bone density test (a painless test that is the only true way to diagnose the condition), and take charge!

The prevention and management of osteoporosis involves attention to nutrition, possible use of medication, and physical exercise. For your nutritional needs, I suggest that you consult a dietitian or nutritionist; for questions on medication or medical management, consult a physician who specializes in osteoporosis. For exercise, follow the program in this book.

My program has three important differences from other programs:

1. The exercises are site-specific. Emphasis is placed on (a) strengthening the back extensors, the deep layer of back muscles that hold the body up against the force of gravity (muscles neglected in most exercise programs), and (b) stretching certain areas to restore normal body alignment.

2. The exercises are safe for nearly everyone. There are no sit-ups, straight leg raises, toe touches, or knee-to-chest movements *(see sidebar)*. Research has shown that these types of exercises should not be performed by people with fragile bones because fracture risk is greatly increased.*

3. The exercises start at a low level. You begin by lying on your back to take compression off the vertebral column, continuing on to isometric strengthening and flexibility.

Start today! You will be on your way to improved posture, relief of back pain, and prevention of the devastating effects of osteoporosis. Although it is never too late to begin, the earlier you start the better.

Sara Meeks

---

* Sinaki, M & Mikkelsen, BA (1988). Postmenopausal spinal osteoporosis: flexion vs extension exercises. *Archives Physical Medicine and Rehab., 69:277-80.*

Info @ aapmr. org.

INTRODUCTION

Most back pain is caused by poor posture, faulty body mechanics, and weak back musculature, which are the result of a lifetime of habits formed as we go about our daily routine.

Most of what we do is in front of us, therefore we develop tightness in areas that pull us forward and weakness in areas that pull us backward.

Correcting posture, following good body mechanics, and strengthening your back can eliminate back pain.

THIS IS THE PROGRAM for postural correction and muscle strengthening that I developed for my patients with osteoporosis. Done correctly and consistently, it can relieve pain, improve body alignment, and restore some body height. (The same program can also help people who have back and neck pain from other causes, such as slipped disk, degenerative disc disease, spondylolisthesis, etc.).

There are six parts to the Meeks' Osteoporosis Program:

MENTAL IMAGERY (Chapter I) will get you off to a good start because you will see a difference in posture almost immediately. At first the visualizations may seem difficult because you are not used to combining mind and body effort (for example, are you aware of your posture as you read this?). Practice the visualizations frequently as you go about your daily activities.

SITE-SPECIFIC EXERCISES (Chapter II) strengthen the muscles needed for good posture and relief of spinal compression and stretch areas that need more flexibility to assist in a return to good body alignment. They should be performed at a regular time each day.

BALANCE (Chapter III) training reduces your risk of falling. You will learn how to assess your balance and to perform specific exercises to maintain or improve balance.

WALKING (Chapter IV) in good alignment is a weightbearing exercise that is unparalleled in its simplicity and effectiveness. Begin walking at the same time as you begin the entire program.

SCAPULAR STABILIZATION (Chapter V) is important for good body alignment. If you have a history of a shoulder or arm injury and are having pain and weakness, you may have to wait until you have acquired the shoulder flexibility and back strength to tolerate the exercises. Otherwise they can usually be started by the third or fourth exercise session.

GOOD BODY MECHANICS (Chapter VI) are essential for the prevention and treatment of osteoporosis and back pain. Any exercise program will be ineffective unless it is accompanied by the practice of good body mechanics during your daily activities.

❧

When you begin the program, make a commitment to follow it for 4 to 6 weeks. During this period, discontinue any other exercises you may be doing. Except where specifically indicated, you need to perform the entire program to get the full benefit.

As your body alignment changes, you may find that maintaining your new posture makes you tire easily. That should be only temporary. Your muscles and ligaments have become stretched and weakened from years of poor postural habits, and your body will need time to get used to its new positioning and to gain the back strength for holding your new body alignment.

Commitment raises energy to a high level because it eliminates indecision.

Be patient. Soon you will have less fatigue and muscle soreness, your new body alignment will become more of a habit, and your friends will wonder why you look so different. As 81-year old Natalie Light of Gainesville, Florida, exclaimed, *"I always feel 5 pounds thinner and 2 inches taller when I finish my exercise session!"*

CHAPTER I

MENTAL IMAGERY

"YES, YOU CAN BE TALLER!"

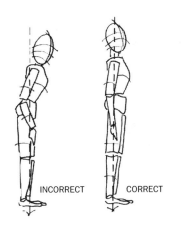

INCORRECT   CORRECT

GOOD BODY ALIGNMENT CAN MAKE a big difference in your life. It can make you be taller, look better, breathe better, have less pain, and improve digestion and elimination. Good postural habits can be learned even after many years of poor habits. Conscious effort and time are required, but the rewards are truly worthwhile.

When you follow these four visualizations, you should see your posture change almost immediately. Practice them when you walk, when you stand and when you sit. They will gradually become easier to remember and more of a habit.

1. DROP AN IMAGINARY PLUMB LINE

If a straight line were dropped beside your body from the ceiling to the floor, and you were in good body alignment, that line would pass through your ear, shoulder, hip, knee and ankle *(see figure at left)*.

Picture this line, and the next three visualizations, no matter what you are doing. Correct your body alignment right then and there.

2. THINK TALLER

Most of us do not stand or sit up to our full height. We are used to slouching, allowing our head and shoulders to fall forward and our rib cage to approach our pelvis. These images will help you straighten up and make you taller.

Pretend you are 2" taller than you are (or any height you want to be, or used to be).

Pretend that a rope hanging from the ceiling is attached to the crown of your head, pulling you up as if you were a puppet (do not tilt your head back).

Pretend that someone is holding you by the scruff of your neck (at the base

*It will not help to work on just
one part of your body. For example,
most people who pull their shoulders
back to "straighten the plumb line"
also pull their elbows back;
that motion makes their head and
shoulders go forward, and may
result, several years later, in much
worsened alignment: the so-called
"grasshopper" posture.*

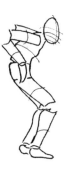

of the skull) and is pulling you up by lengthening your back.

Pretend that another rope is attached to your breastbone, lifting your rib cage.

Women: imagine you have a fine jewel that rests on the notch where your collarbones come together and you want to show it off; lift and be proud of your breasts (many women have poor posture stemming from self-consciousness when they were developing in adolescence; it is time to change that old habit). Men: keep your necktie high ("tie-high").

3. KEEP YOUR PELVIS LEVEL

Place your hands on your waist (actually the top of your pelvic bones). Pretend your pelvis is a bucket and you must keep the bucket level.

Depending on how you stand, you may have to tuck your tailbone under or stick it out (most people need to tuck it under). Either movement will begin to strengthen your abdominal and back muscles as they isometrically contract to hold the "bucket" position.

4. LENGTHEN YOUR MID-SECTION

With both hands, feel the top of your pelvic bones ("hip bones"); then feel the bottom of your rib cage. Now lift your upper body and increase the space between your rib cage and pelvis.

CHAPTER II

SITE-SPECIFIC EXERCISES

These exercises are safe, even if you have severe discomfort or deformity, loss of body height, or compression fractures.

AS WE LIVE our daily lives, we develop habits and patterns of movement that increase our efficiency. At the expense of this efficiency, imbalances in muscular and joint function result which can cause changes in body alignment and pain. Eventually, our ability to carry out our daily activities is affected, and we may have problems with balance. All of this puts us at risk for serious injury.

The age-old admonition to "stand up straight" does not work to change this situation. To effect a permanent change, some structures need to be stretched and others need to be strengthened.

The exercises in this chapter are "site-specific" in two important ways: 1) they directly target the prime areas of restriction and weakness. And 2), they increase a bone's density by contracting (and thus strengthening) the muscles that attach to that bone (such as the spinal vertebrae). The exercises that perform this function are identified by a bone symbol (✐).

HOW OFTEN SHOULD YOU EXERCISE?

If your bones are strong enough, one session daily should be sufficient. But if you have osteoporosis or have any of the signs of osteoporosis (lost body height or compression fractures, for example), exercising 2 or 3 times a day would be better in the beginning. After four to six weeks, you could (depending on your condition) decrease the frequency and maintain the benefits.

HOW LONG SHOULD YOU EXERCISE AT A TIME?

That will depend on your physical condition. Start at the beginning, and stop when you feel tired. You will eventually build up the muscles and strength to continue through the entire program. A complete exercise session will take 30 to 45 minutes.

IS IT BETTER TO DO MORE REPETITIONS THAN SUGGESTED?

No. Because the exercises are site-specific, you don't need many repetitions. You will benefit from an exercise by doing it completely and in good form just a few times.

SHOULD THE EXERCISES BE DONE IN THE ORDER GIVEN?

The standing exercises can be done at any time, and you will find they make you feel better in many situations. They are particularly effective for relief of back strain, such as after sitting for a long time or bending slightly forward (as when doing the dishes).

The others should be followed in order because they build on one another. As you gain strength and become familiar with the program, you can skip those that build to more difficult versions (these are noted in the text). On days when you are feeling stiff or sore or tired, you can return to the easier versions.

LYING ON YOUR BACK: KNEES STRAIGHT OR BENT?

When you begin the program, I want you to lie on your back with your knees bent, feet flat on the floor and pointing straight ahead, feet and knees hip distance apart. In this position, the shoulder and head exercises are easier to do, back strain is relieved, and most excess lumbar lordosis (space between the floor and low back) is relieved. Later, if you have no strain or discomfort in your back, you can lie on your back with legs extended and knees straight.

DO YOU HAVE TO LIE ON THE FLOOR?

For the most benefit, exercises (except standing ones) are best done on the floor, on a carpet or mat. If you have a balance problem or any physical limitation that would make it difficult or unsafe to get down and up from the floor, you can exercise on your bed. Later, as you get stronger, you can change to the floor.

MUSCLE SORENESS

It is natural to have sore muscles, especially in the mid-back and calf areas, as you use "new" muscles. Any soreness should be temporary and relieved by a hot shower, moist heating pad, massage or ice pack. But do not be concerned if you have no soreness; that is natural, too.

WHAT IF AN OLD INJURY STARTS BOTHERING YOU?

As your postural alignment begins to change, symptoms of an old injury, or a condition for which you had surgery, may return. For example, it is common for an old knee injury to resurface.

Do not be discouraged. In all likelihood, the old injury did not heal in good alignment. Perhaps it was not treated or, even if it was, there may have been some residual limitation of motion or loss of strength and you have compensated (subconsciously) for the limitation by a change in body alignment, with resultant back pain. Now, as the back and pelvis become re-aligned, you may experience recurrent knee pain. If the problem persists, you may need to work with a physical therapist for specific exercises, heat or cold treatment, or massage to the area.

WHAT IF YOU ARE "STUCK" AND NOT IMPROVING?

You may have specific areas with limitation. For example, a goal with the Arm Lengthener *(page 30)* is to comfortably straighten your arms alongside your head. If you have been working diligently on such a movement with no improvement, you may need to work with a physical therapist to increase your range of motion.

BREATHING WHILE YOU EXERCISE: VERY IMPORTANT!

Pay attention to your breathing patterns as you exercise. Breathe OUT as you hold a muscle contraction or stretch. Do not hold your breath. In general, keep your breathing relaxed.

Each time you perform the first exercise, follow this breathing "warm-up." Breathe deeply for a few minutes using your abdominal muscles. Place your hands lightly on your belly. Breathe in, allowing your belly to expand and push against your hands, then breathe out, pulling the belly in (push gently with your hands). Imagine there is a balloon in your belly; blow it up as you breathe in and deflate it as you breathe out.

THE FIRST EXERCISE: THE DECOMPRESSION EXERCISE

Turn to page 20 and look at The Decompression Exercise. It may not seem like an exercise at all, but it is! Lying on your back helps straighten the curves of the back, it relieves compression of the vertebral bodies, and it helps the back to relax. In addition to being an exercise in and of itself, it is the starting position for other exercises that help strengthen the back.

You may wonder, how long is it useful to "just lie there"? The answer varies, according to your circumstances.

o *If you do not have osteopenia or osteoporosis (or any back problem at all):* The exercise is helpful at the end of the day after hours of sitting and standing. Stay in the position at least 1 minute.

o *If you have a back condition such as a slipped disc or spondylolisthesis:* Do the exercise several times each day and stay in position at least 5 minutes.

o *If you have osteopenia or mild osteoporosis:* Even if you are not having back pain or do not have any of the postural changes associated with osteoporosis, you should lie on your back at least once a day for 5 to 15 minutes.

o *If you have severe osteoporosis with postural changes:* You should lie on your back at least once a day (but preferably 3–5 times a day) for 5 to 15 minutes. Your goal is to be able to lie on your back comfortably, with knees straight and no pillow under your head. Be very patient; this may take several weeks or even months to accomplish, especially if you have not been able to lie on your back for several years. If you have a dowager's hump, you may always need some kind of support, especially for your head.

THE DECOMPRESSION EXERCISE

Body position is very important for this exercise. Follow the instructions carefully, and use the same supports (pillow, etc.) for the other exercises that start from this position.

1. **Lie on your back with knees bent, feet flat on floor and pointing straight ahead. Knees and feet hip distance apart.**

   Your face should be parallel to the floor. Have someone look at you from the side to make sure that your head is not too far forward (chin toward chest) or backward (chin pointing upward).

   If your head is tilted back, place a pillow or folded towel under it. You may also need a pillow under your shoulders. (A tilted-back head is most frequently associated with an exaggerated thoracic kyphosis that results in forward shoulders and head.)

   If your head is tilted forward, place a towel roll under your *NECK*.

2. **Arms at sides, slightly away from body, palms up.**

   Your elbows and shoulders should be at the same level. If your shoulders are higher than your elbows, place support under your elbows.

3. **Stay in this position 1–5 minutes.**

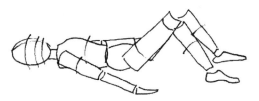

This exercise (1) increases tolerance for lying on your back; (2) helps align the curves of the back; (3) relieves compression of the vertebral bodies; (4) helps the back to relax.

SHOULDER PRESS

1. **Lie on your back as in the Decompression Exercise** *(page 20)*.

2. **Press shoulders downward toward the floor.**

   If it is difficult to press both shoulders at the same time, press one at a time and work up to being able to press both shoulders at the same time. It may also be helpful to move your arms farther away from your body.
   (Breathe out as you press your shoulders back. Do not hold your breath.)

3. **Hold 2–3 seconds, then relax.**

   Do not "hunch" your shoulders toward your ears. Do not arch your lower back and do not "roll" your arms; keep all the motion in the shoulders.

4. **Repetitions: 3–5.**

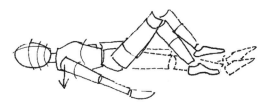

This exercise (1) strengthens the muscles between the shoulder blades; (2) strengthens the muscles that extend the spine and hold your back straight against the force of gravity; (3) stretches the muscles on the front of the shoulders and chest, thus helping to correct a rounded or forward shoulder posture; (4) relieves compression of the vertebral bodies.

CHIN TUCK/ HEAD SLIDE/ HEAD PRESS

If you placed a towel under your NECK in the Decompression Exercise, do not do the chin tuck/head slide; do just the head press.

If you placed a towel under your HEAD, begin with the chin tuck/head slide. Later, as your neck muscles begin to stretch, you will also be able to do the Head Press.

1. **Lie on your back as in the Decompression Exercise** *(page 20).*

2. **Tuck chin SLIGHTLY toward your chest** *(see sidebar).*

    When you tuck your chin properly, your mouth remains closed and your entire head slides slightly on the floor. Feel the back of your neck lengthening.

3. **With your chin tucked and neck lengthened, press the back of your head downward into the floor (or pillow, towel, etc.)**

    Do not tilt your head back as you press it down. Touch the back of your neck lightly with your fingertips and feel the neck muscles contract.
    (Breathe out during entire tuck/press movement.)

4. **Hold 2–3 seconds, then relax.**

    Important: Start this exercise gently.

5. **Repetitions: 3–5.**

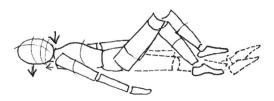

This exercise (1) helps re-align the head over the shoulders; (2) strengthens the muscles that hold the head up against the force of gravity; (3) stretches the muscles on the front of the neck.

LEG LENGTHENER

If you feel tightness, muscle cramping or low back discomfort, omit this exercise, and do the Leg Lengthener Variations on the next page instead.

1. **Lie on your back as in the Decompression Exercise *(page 20)*.**

2. **Straighten right leg down to the floor. Pull toes and forefoot toward the knee and extend the heel; "lengthen" leg by pulling your hip away from your rib cage.**

   The lengthening movement should occur in the lower back.
   (Breathe out as you lengthen your leg. Do not hold your breath.)

3. **Hold 2–3 seconds, then relax. Repeat 1 time, then re-bend your knee.**

4. **Repeat #2 and #3 with the left leg.**

5. **Repetitions: 2–3 (total of 4–6 lengtheners with each leg).**

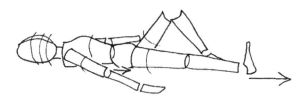

This exercise (1) stretches the heel cord, calf musculature, muscles on the front of the hip joint and muscles of the lower back; (2) strengthens the buttocks muscles, the muscles on the front of the knee, and the muscles that pick up your foot when you walk.

LEG LENGTHENER VARIATIONS

If you start with these variations, you may return to the complete Leg Lengthener exercise (page 23) when your symptoms subside.

LEG STRAIGHTENER

1. **Lie on your back as in the Decompression Exercise** *(page 20).*

2. **Straighten right leg down to the floor; hold position 2–3 seconds; re-bend knee, and repeat 1 time.**
   (Breathe out as you straighten your leg.)

3. **Repeat #2 with the left leg.**

4. **Repeat sequence (right leg, then left leg) for a total of 4–6 "straighteners" with each leg.**

HEEL EXTENDER

1. **Lie on your back as in the Decompression Exercise (page 20).**

2. **Straighten right leg down to the floor. Pull toes and forefoot toward the knee and extend the heel. Hold position 2–3 seconds, then relax foot.**
   (Breathe out as you extend your heel.)

3. **Repeat foot motion 1 time. Re-bend knee.**

4. **Repeat #2 and #3 with the left leg.**

5. **Repeat sequence (right leg, then left leg) for a total of 4–6 heel extenders with each leg.**

BUTTOCK SQUEEZE

1. **Lie on your back with legs extended, hip distance apart, feet relaxed.**

   A small pillow may be placed under your knees to reduce strain on the lower back.

2. **Arms at sides, palms up, slightly away from the body, or resting on abdomen.**

   With arms at sides, your elbows should be at the same level as your shoulders.

3. **Squeeze buttocks muscles as tightly as possible (say: "tight, tighter, tightest") and lift tailbone slightly off the floor. Hold 2–3 seconds, then relax.**

   (Breathe out as you contract and hold the buttocks.)

4. **Repetitions: 3–5.**

If this muscle group is weak, you may have difficulty isolating it. To contract the correct muscles, pretend you are about to have a bowel movement and have to hold it.

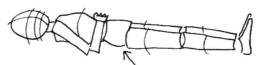

This exercise (1) stretches the muscles on the front of the hip; (2) strengthens the buttocks, lower back musculature, and upper hamstrings.

LEG PRESS

When you are comfortable exercising one leg at a time, do the exercise with both legs at the same time.

1. **Lie on your back as in the Decompression Exercise** *(page 20).*

2. **Straighten right leg down to the floor, pull toes and forefoot toward the knee, extend the heel and press the entire leg downward.**

   Imagine you are lying on the beach and want to leave an indentation of your leg in the sand. *(Breathe out as you press your leg down.)*

3. **Hold 2–3 seconds, then relax. Repeat. Re-bend the knee.**

4. **Repeat #2 and #3 with the left leg.**

5. **Repetitions: 4–6 presses with each leg.**

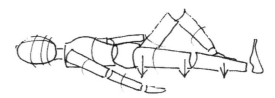

This exercise (1) stretches the muscles on the front of the hip, the heel cord, calf muscles, and the tendons at the back of the knee; (2) strengthens the buttocks, upper hamstrings, lower back, the muscles on the front of the knee, and the muscles that pick up your foot when you walk.

ANKLE PUMPS/ CALF STRETCH

1. **Lie on your back as in the Decompression Exercise *(page 20)*.**

   If you prefer you may sit with your back supported.

2. **Straighten right leg down to the floor.**

3. **With your knee straight, "pump" your right ankle: pull toes and forefoot up toward the knee and then push toes and forefoot away from the knee.**

   Emphasize heel movement—push your heel away as your toes move upward; pull heel upward as toes and forefoot move downward. If you are seated, straighten your knee first, then "pump" your ankle. *(Keep breathing relaxed.)*

4. **Repeat #2 and #3 with the left leg.**

5. **Repetitions: 10–15 times with each ankle.**

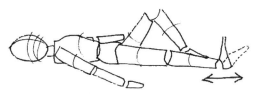

This exercise (1) helps increase flexibility of the ankle joint; (2) helps relieve swelling of the ankles and lower legs, thus helping to improve circulation and relieve night cramps.

ELBOW PRESS

1. **Lie on your back as in the Decompression Exercise** *(page 20).*

2. **Interlace your fingers; bring your arms up and place your hands underneath your head (not under your neck).**

   If you cannot get your hands behind your head, bring them to your forehead or to the top of your head. As you gain flexibility, work toward getting them behind your head.

3. **Press elbows downward and outward, toward the floor. Hold 2–3 seconds, then relax.**

   Do not bring elbows together between presses. *(Breathe out as you press.)*

   If your elbows do not reach the floor or if the movement causes pain in your shoulders, place a pillow or folded towel on the floor under your elbows, and press your elbows against this support.

4. **Repetitions: 3–5.**

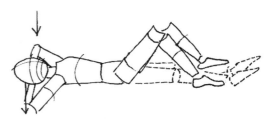

This exercise (1) strengthens the muscles between the shoulder blades; (2) stretches the muscles across the front of the shoulders and chest, thus helping to correct a rounded or forward shoulder posture.

THORACIC LIFT

Builds on Shoulder Press

Omit this exercise until you can do the Shoulder Press (page 21) with both shoulders.

1. **Lie on your back as in the Decompression Exercise *(page 20)*.**

2. **Press both shoulders down toward the floor; keeping your shoulders pressed back, lift your mid-back (between shoulder blades) off the floor.**

   Press harder than you did with the Shoulder Press. *(Breathe out as you press and lift.)*

   Important: Shoulders remain pressed back. Emphasize the movement between your shoulder blades. Do not try to arch your lower back; but if it arches slightly as you lift your mid-back, that is OK.

3. **Hold 2–3 seconds, then relax.**

4. **Repetitions: 3–5.**

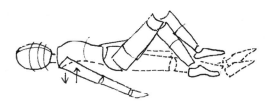

This exercise (1) strengthens the muscles between the shoulder blades; (2) strengthens the long back extensor muscles that hold the back straight against the force of gravity; (3) stretches the muscles across the front of the shoulders and chest; (4) relieves compression of the vertebral bodies in the thoracic spine, helping to reduce thoracic kyphosis (dowager's hump).

ARM LENGTHENER

When you are able to rest your arms comfortably on the floor alongside your head, many daily activities that involve reaching will become easier.

After you are comfortable moving one arm at a time, you can do the exercise with both arms at the same time.

1. **Lie on your back as in the Decompression Exercise** *(page 20)*.

2. **Arms at sides, palms down.**

3. **Flatten your lower back against the floor by contracting your abdominal and buttocks muscles ("set" your pelvis).**

4. **Keep elbow straight, and bring right arm up over your head as far as you can. "Lengthen" arm by pulling rib cage up and away from your pelvis.**

   If one arm is painful, it may help to hold a cane or stick in both hands and move both arms together; your stronger arm will assist the weaker, painful one. *(Breathe out as you lengthen your arm.)*

5. **Hold 2–3 seconds, then relax with arm still in "up" position. "Lengthen" arm again, then return it to your side.**

6. **Repeat #4 and #5 with left arm.**

7. **Repetitions: 4–6 "lengtheners" for each arm.**

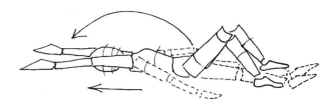

This exercise (1) increases shoulder range of motion (to decrease stress and prevent injury to the back during reaching); (2) stretches the muscles along the sides of the body between the rib cage and pelvis.

COVER THE BONES

Builds on Shoulder Press and the Thoracic Lift)

You will need to master both the Shoulder Press (page 21) and the Thoracic Lift (page 29) before you are able to do this exercise well.

1. **Lie on your back as in the Decompression Exercise** *(page 20).*

2. **Press both shoulders down toward the floor, and lift your mid-back (between the shoulder blades) off the floor.**

   Press and lift harder than you did with the Thoracic Lift. *(Breathe out as you press and lift.)*

   Do not arch your lower back. Imagine you are tucking your spine into a group of muscles that run up and down your back, so that the muscles cover the spine.

3. **Hold 2–3 seconds, then relax.**

4. **Repetitions: 3–5.**

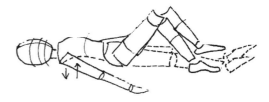

This exercise (1) strengthens the muscles between the shoulder blades; (2) strengthens the long back extensor muscles that hold you up against the force of gravity; (3) stretches the muscles across the front of the shoulders and chest; (4) relieves compression of the vertebral bodies in the thoracic spine, helping to reduce thoracic kyphosis (dowager's hump).

MORNING STRETCHES

Combines Leg Lengthener and Arm Lengthener

When you can do Leg Lengtheners (page 23) and Arm Lengtheners (page 30) without discomfort, you can skip them and go directly to this exercise.

1. Lie on your back with legs extended, hip distance apart, knees straight, feet relaxed.

2. Arms at sides, palms down.

3. Keep elbows straight as you bring both arms up and back over your head as far as you can.

4. With both feet, pull toes and forefeet toward knees, and extend heels.

5. Keeping your arms back and feet pulled up, stretch and "lengthen":

   a. right arm/right leg; hold 2–3 seconds, then relax.

   b. left arm/left leg; hold 2–3 seconds, then relax.

   c. right arm/left leg; hold 2–3 seconds, then relax.

   d. left arm/right leg; hold 2–3 seconds, then relax.

   e. both arms/both legs; hold 2–3 seconds, then relax.

   As you stretch, concentrate on increasing the space between rib cage and pelvis. *(Breathe out as you stretch. Do not hold your breath.)*

6. Repetitions: 1–2 for each movement.

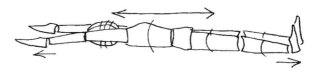

This exercise (1) increases flexibility of shoulders and ankles; (2) stretches the muscles between the rib cage and pelvis, thereby lengthening the mid-section of the body.

ARM PRESS

1. **Lie on your back as in the Decompression Exercise** *(page 20)*.

2. **Arms at sides, palms down.**

3. **Keep elbow straight, and bring right arm up and back over your head until it rests on the floor alongside your head.**

   If your arm does not reach the floor, place a pillow or folded towel on the floor so your arm can rest on it. Your arm MUST have something to press against.

4. **Press arm into floor. Hold 2–3 seconds, then relax. Repeat 1 time. Return arm to your side.**

   (Breathe out as you press arm down.)

5. **Repeat #4 and #5 with left arm.**

6. **Then repeat with both arms together. Repeat 1 time.**

7. **Repeat entire sequence (#4–#7) 1 time.**

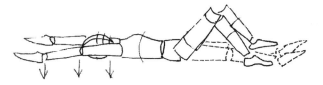

This exercise (1) strengthens the lower trapezius, a muscle at the bottom of the shoulder blade that pulls the shoulder blade downward and backward; (2) stabilizes the shoulder girdle during shoulder joint movement, thereby helping prevent rotator cuff injuries.

ANGELS IN THE SNOW

Pretend you are lying in the snow and want to leave an impression of your arm movement ("angel wings"). Your arms should remain on the floor as you move them, with palms turned up.

1. **Lie on your back as in the Decompression Exercise *(page 20)*.**

2. **Arms on floor, palms up: slide right arm out to the side and up over your head; when you reach as far as you can, "lengthen" arm, then relax. "Lengthen" again, and return arm to your side (palm up, arm on floor).**

   As you slide your arm out, you may feel a good "pull." You should not feel pain. *(Breathe out as you lengthen your arm.)*

3. **Repeat with left arm.**

4. **Repeat with both arms at the same time.**

   If you have full range of motion (arms resting beside head, elbows straight) and find it easy to reach that position with one arm at a time, you can omit that part and move both arms together. But if you have limitation of motion in either shoulder, continue moving each arm separately.

5. **Repetitions: 1**

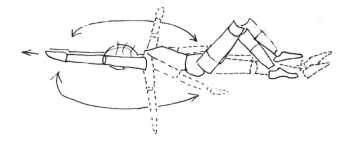

This exercise (1) increases shoulder flexibility; (2) stretches the mid-back, especially when both arms move at the same time; (3) stretches the muscles across front of shoulders and chest.

This exercise is strenuous. Follow instructions precisely. Keep your buttocks tight and lift buttocks and back only as far as you can without pain or cramping. DO NOT HOLD YOUR BREATH when your body is in the lifted position; that can raise blood pressure.

BRIDGING (4 VARIATIONS)

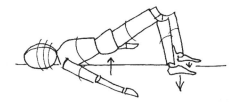

1. **Lie on your back as in the Decompression Exercise** *(page 20).*
2. **Arms at sides, elbows straight, palms down.**
3. **Press down on feet, squeeze buttocks together, press down on arms, gradually tuck and lift tailbone, then buttocks, lower, mid and upper back. Hold 2–3 seconds.** * *(Breathe evenly as you move and throughout the hold.)*
4. **Gently return upper, mid, lower back, then buttocks to floor. Relax.**
5. **Repetitions: 1–2.**

   If you have cramping of muscles on back of thigh or lower back pain, try this instead: press down on feet, hold 2–3 seconds and relax. Repeat 3–5 times. Gradually try to contract buttocks, lift tailbone, etc. as you are able to tolerate it.

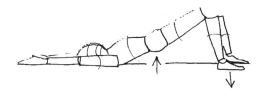

1. **Lie on your back as in the Decompression Exercise** *(page 20).*
2. **Arms alongside your head, resting on or near the floor, with elbows straight and palms up,**
3. **Press down on feet, squeeze buttocks together, gradually tuck and lift tailbone, then buttocks, lower, mid and upper back. Hold 2–3 seconds.** *
   (Breathe evenly as you move and throughout the hold.)
4. **Gently return upper, mid, lower back, then buttocks to floor. Relax.**
5. **Repetitions: 1–2.**

* If you can, work up to holding 30 seconds; later, you may progress to several minutes.

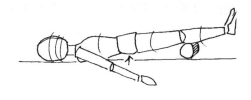

1. Lie on your back, knees bent over a foam roller or large pillow.
2. Arms at sides, palms down.
3. Raise both feet up by straightening knees; gradually tuck and lift tailbone, then buttocks, lower, mid- and upper back off the floor. Hold 2–3 seconds. *
   (Breathe evenly throughout the hold.)
4. Gently return upper, mid-, lower back, then buttocks to floor. Relax.
5. Repetitions: 1–2.

* *If you can, work up to 30 seconds; later, you may progress to several minutes.*

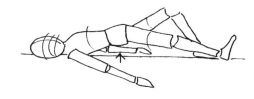

1. Lie on your back as in the Decompression Exercise *(page 20)*.
2. Arms at sides, palms down.
3. Press down on feet, squeeze buttocks together, press down on arms, gradually tuck and lift tailbone, then buttocks, lower, mid- and upper back.
4. Keeping hips level, slide right foot out so that only the heel is on floor; keep buttocks tight and back as high as possible. Hold 2–3 seconds, then return leg to starting position. *(Breathe evenly throughout the hold.)*
5. Repeat #4 with left leg.
6. Gently return upper, mid-, lower back, then buttocks to floor. Relax.
7. Repetitions: 1–2.

This exercise (1) strengthens some of the major muscles of the body, including buttocks, abdominals, and back extensors; (2) stretches the muscles on front of hips and knees.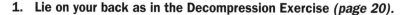

THE CAT

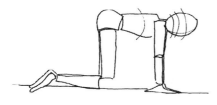

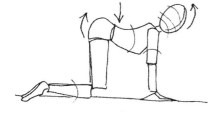

IF YOU DO NOT HAVE OSTEOPOROSIS, you can do both parts, alternating between them without pausing in the "table" position.

1. **Get onto your hands and knees. Your back should be flat, with hands under shoulders, knees under hips, and body weight evenly distributed.**

   Imagine your back is a table and your arms and legs are the legs of the table.

2. **Lift tailbone, allowing lower back then mid and upper back to "sag."**

   Keep elbows straight and weight even between hands and knees. All movement is in the spine; it starts at the tailbone, and "rolls" up the back.

3. **Raise head and look upward; hold 2–3 seconds.** *(Breathe out while raising head.)*

4. **Return to starting (table) position by tucking your tailbone, flattening your back and lowering your head.**

5. **Repetitions: 1–5.**

This exercise (1) increases flexibility of the vertebral column; (2) strengthens the arms.

DO NOT DO THE FOLLOWING MOVEMENTS IF YOU HAVE OSTEOPOROSIS (if in doubt, have a bone density test), and especially if you have a dowager's hump, because these movements place too much flexion force on the spine.

1. **Get onto hands and knees as above.**

2. **Tuck tailbone; round lower, mid and upper back.**

3. **Lower head between your arms.**

   (Breathe out as you are lowering your head.)

4. **Return to starting (table) position.**

5. **Repetitions: 1–5.**

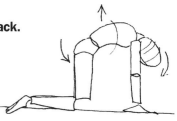

SHOULDER RETRACTION

1. **Stand with good body alignment, with your feet hip distance apart and pointed straight ahead. (You may sit if you like.)**

   See page 13 for description of good body alignment.

2. **Interlace your fingers behind your back, keeping elbows straight.**

   If it is a strain to interlace your fingers, grasp a cane or washcloth with your hands.

3. **Squeeze your backbone with your shoulder blades.**

   (Breathe out as you squeeze and hold.)

   Do not thrust your head forward.
   Do not "hunch" your shoulders toward your ears.
   Do not arch your lower back.
   Do not move your hands away from your body.
   The movement is all in the shoulders.

4. **Hold 2–3 seconds, then relax.**

5. **Repetitions: 3–5.**

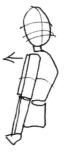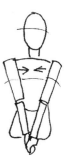

This is a particularly good exercise to do after sitting for a long time.

This exercise (1) strengthens the muscles between the shoulder blades; (2) stretches the muscles across the front of the shoulders and chest, to help correct rounded shoulders.

SHOULDER RETRACTION WITH DEPRESSION

Builds on Shoulder Retraction

1. **Stand with good body alignment, with your feet hip distance apart and pointed straight ahead.**

2. **Interlace your fingers behind your back, keeping elbows straight.**

3. **Squeeze your backbone with your shoulder blades. Hold position, and pull shoulders slightly downward and lift chest slightly.**

Keep shoulder blades together as you pull shoulders downward.
(Breathe out as you squeeze and pull shoulders down.)

The movement is all in the shoulders.
Do not move your arms away from your body.
Do not thrust your head forward.
Do not "hunch" your shoulders toward your ears.
Do not arch your lower back.

4. **Hold 2–3 seconds, then relax.**

5. **Repetitions: 3–5.**

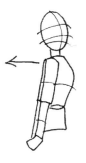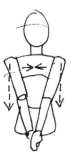

This is a particularly good exercise to do after sitting for a long time.

This exercise (1) strengthens the muscles between the shoulder blades; (2) stretches the muscles across the front of the shoulders and chest, by so doing, helps correct a rounded or forward shoulder posture.

EXTENSION-IN-STANDING

1. **Stand with good body alignment, with your feet hip distance apart and pointed straight ahead.**

2. **Hands on waist with thumbs facing forward.**

3. **Squeeze buttocks and gently press hips forward over knees.**

   (Breathe out as you squeeze and press hips.)

   Important:
   > Do not bend your knees.
   > Do not do a pelvic tilt.
   > Do not arch your upper back.

4. **Hold 2–3 seconds, then relax.**

5. **Repetitions: 3–5.**

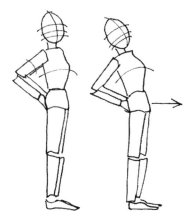

This is a particularly good exercise to do after sitting for a long time.

This exercise (1) strengthens the buttocks muscles; (2) stretches the muscles in the front of the hips, shoulders, and chest.

PUSHAWAYS

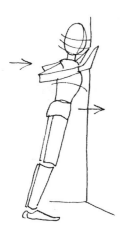

1. **Stand facing a wall (or corner or doorway).**

   Facing a wall is the easiest position. The corner and doorway are more difficult.

2. **Place hands on wall at shoulder height, a little farther apart than your shoulders, fingers pointed upward.**

3. **Keep your body absolutely straight, elbows up, and lean into the wall.**

   Your heels should stay on the floor. If your heels come up, move closer to the wall. Your body should be "like a board" and should not bend anywhere except at your elbows, wrists, and ankles.

   (Keep breathing normal and even; you can breathe out either as you approach the wall, or as you push away.)

4. **Hold position 2–3 seconds, then push away with your arms.**

5. **Repetitions: 2–3.**

This is similar to a military push-up, done in a standing position. It is a particularly good exercise to do after sitting for a long time.

This exercise (1) strengthens the muscles between the shoulder blades and the muscles of the arms; (2) strengthens the arms (it is a good beginning weightbearing exercise for the arms); (3) stretches the heel cords; (4) stretches the muscles across the front of the shoulders and chest.

The next group of exercises involves lying on the abdomen, with head straight and forehead resting on your hands, palms down. If the position is uncomfortable, you may need to spend 2 or 3 sessions getting used to it. You may want a small pillow or rolled towel under your forehead. A pillow may also be placed under the hips and/or chest, and a roll under the ankles to prevent pressure on toes or front of feet.

BELLY PRESS

The Belly Press position is important for exercises done on the abdomen because you can lift the legs, arch the back and complete other body movements more easily and safely.

1. **Lie on abdomen, head straight, with forehead resting on hands, palms down (starting position).**

2. **Now place hands, palms up, under your prominent front hip bones.**

3. **Rest your head on forehead or chin. If you have a problem breathing, place a small towel or pillow under forehead.**

4. **Press your pelvic and abdominal area into the floor.**

   This is a pressing of the body into the floor to stabilize the pelvis. It is not a pelvic tilt—do not lift the abdomen. *(Breathe out as you press and hold.)*

   Your legs may begin to lift slightly off the floor and you may notice some extension of your back. Do not try to move your legs or back; just press the front of your body into the floor.

5. **Hold 2–3 seconds, then relax.**

6. **Repetitions: 3–5.**

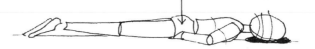

This exercise strengthens the buttocks, upper hamstrings and lower back extensors (muscles that straighten your back and help hold your body up against the force of gravity).

ALTERNATE HIP EXTENSION

1. **Lie on your abdomen, hands under hip bones or arms at your sides, palms UP, with head straight, resting on forehead or chin.**

   Head straight—not turned to the side.

2. **Press your pelvic and abdominal area into the floor (Belly Press).**

3. **Lifting from hip and keeping knee straight, raise and lengthen your left leg.**

   Lift leg straight up (toward ceiling). Press opposite leg into floor to help stabilize the body. Do not twist your body. *(Breathe out as you lift your leg.)*

4. **Hold 2–3 seconds, then relax. Repeat 1 time.**

5. **Repeat with right leg.**

6. **Repetitions: 2–3 (total leg lifts for each leg).**

   You can also lift both legs together. If you have weakness of one leg, however, be sure to lift each leg separately as well as both together.

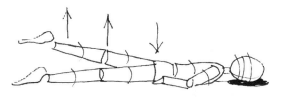

This exercise (1) strengthens the large hip extensors (buttocks and upper hamstrings); (2) strengthens the lower back extensors that help hold the back up against the force of gravity.

SHOULDER BLADE SQUEEZE

5 VARIATIONS

1. **Lie on your abdomen, arms alongside body, elbows straight, palms up. Head straight, resting on forehead or chin.**

2. **Press your pelvic and abdominal area into the floor (Belly Press).**

3. **Squeeze backbone with your shoulder blades.**

4. **Keeping your shoulder blades together, raise chest and head.**

   In the first four variations, make sure you actually raise your shoulders and squeeze the shoulder blades together before and as you lift your head and chest.
   (Breathe out as you lift and hold.)

5. **Hold 2–3 seconds, then relax.**

6. **Repetitions: 1–2.**

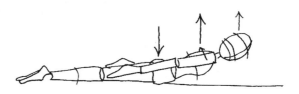

The 5 variations of this exercise (1) strengthen several groups of muscles between the shoulder blades; (2) strengthen the long back extensors (important muscles that hold you up against the force of gravity); (3) stretch the muscles across the front of the chest.

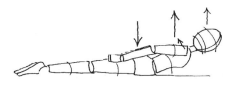

1. Lie on your abdomen, hands interlaced behind low back. Head straight, resting on forehead or chin.

2. Press your pelvic and abdominal area into the floor (Belly Press).

3. Squeeze backbone with shoulder blades; raise front part of shoulders, chest and head from floor *(Breathe out as you lift and hold.)*

4. Hold 2–3 seconds, then relax.

5. Repetitions: 1–2.

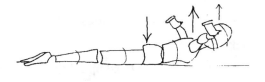

1. Lie on your abdomen, arms straight out to the sides about shoulder level, elbows straight, palms down. Head straight, resting on chin or forehead.

2. Press your pelvic and abdominal area into the floor (Belly Press).

3. Squeeze backbone with shoulder blades as you raise both arms up into "airplane position," keeping elbows straight.

4. Raise chest and head from floor. *(Breathe out as you lift and hold.)*

5. Hold 2–3 seconds. Relax.

6. Repetitions: 1–2.

As you become stronger, progress to the following arm positions. Do not strain, and do not hold your breath.

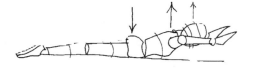

1. **Lie on your abdomen, arms out to the sides at shoulder level. Palms down, elbows bent at a right angle.**
2. **Press your pelvic and abdominal area into the floor (Belly Press).**
3. **Squeeze shoulder blades together as you raise arms from floor.**
4. **Raise chest and head from floor.** *(Breathe out as you lift and hold.)*
5. **Hold 2–3 seconds, then relax.**
6. **Repetitions: 1–2.**

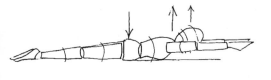

1. **Lie on your abdomen, arms resting on floor extended alongside head, palms down.**
2. **Press your pelvic and abdominal area into the floor (Belly Press).**
3. **Raise both arms by tightening shoulder blade muscles.**
4. **Keep arms close to your ears as you raise chest and head up off the floor.** *(Breathe out as you lift and hold.)*
5. **Hold 2–3 seconds, then relax.**
6. **Repetitions: 1–2.**

HEAD LIFT

This exercise is the same movement as the Head Press (page 22), but since you are lying on your abdomen, it is done against gravity.

1. **Lie on your abdomen, forehead resting on hands, palms down.**

2. **Keep chin tucked and raise head straight up.**

    The actual movement is small, but you must do the exercise correctly so as to get the greatest benefit:

    Do not to tilt your chin as you raise your head.

    Do not raise your shoulders as you raise your head.

    (Breathe out as you lift your head.)

3. **Hold 2–3 seconds, then relax.**

4. **Repetitions: 3–5.**

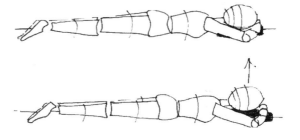

This exercise (1) stretches the tight structures on the front of the neck; (2) strengthens the muscles that hold the head up against the force of gravity.

LEG/ARM LIFT

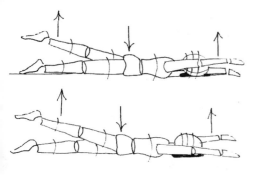

1. Lie on abdomen, arms extended along side of head, palms down. Rest head on forehead or chin.

2. Press pelvic and abdominal area into floor (Belly Press) as you . . .

   a. Lift right arm. Hold 2–3 seconds, then relax.
   b. Lift left arm. Hold 2–3 seconds, then relax.
   c. Lift right leg. Hold 2–3 seconds, then relax.
   d. Lift left leg. Hold 2–3 seconds, then relax.
   e. Lift both arms. Hold 2–3 seconds, then relax.
   f. Lift both legs. Hold 2–3 seconds, then relax.
   g. Lift right arm and left leg. Hold 2–3 seconds, then relax.
   h. Lift left arm and right leg. Hold 2–3 seconds, then relax.
   i. Lift both legs and both arms at the same time. Hold 2–3 seconds, then relax.

   When lifting arms or legs, keep your head down and do not twist your body.
   Raise ARMS from the shoulder, keep them close to your head, with straight elbows.
   Raise LEGS with knees straight; lifting from the hips. *(Breathe out with each lift.)*

3. Repetitions, each position: 1–2.

This exercise strengthens the muscles between the shoulder blades, the strong hip extensors (buttocks, upper hamstrings), and the long back extensors.

THE SPHINX

1. **Lie on your abdomen.**

2. **Prop yourself up on forearms and elbows, palms down, arms shoulder width apart.**

3. **Take slow deep breaths, and feel your stomach sag each time you exhale. Allow your back to relax. Stay in this position at least 3–5 seconds.**

4. **Press elbows into the floor and "pull" back (elbows do not actually move) to feel stretch and traction in your lower back. Keep chest lifted and head in aligment.**

   Pretend you are going to pull your body through your arms, but no movement actually occurs. (*Breathe out as you stretch.*)

5. **Repetitions: 1–2.**

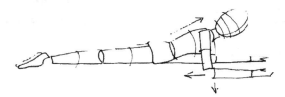

This exercise (1) stretches the muscles on the front on the chest, the abdomen and the front of the hips; (2) is a form of self-traction for the lower back; (3) relieves compression of the thoracic vertebral bodies.

COMBINATION EXERCISE

Combines the movements in the Shoulder Blade Squeezes.

This exercise is strenuous. Be careful not to strain. Keep your chest lifted during all the arm movements, and keep your belly pressed into the floor. If your legs rise from the floor, this is OK, but do not try to raise them.

(Breathe evenly as you hold the positions.)

This exercise is a very powerful strengthener for your back extensors. ✎

50

1. Lie on your abdomen, head resting on forehead or chin.

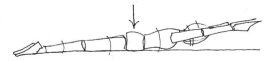

2. Place arms alongside head, elbows straight, palms down, and press pelvic and abdominal area into floor (Belly Press); raise both arms, chest and head. Hold position a few seconds, then . . .

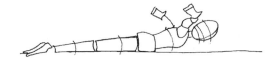

3. Bring your arms out to sides at shoulder level and raise up a little farther. Hold a few seconds, then . . .

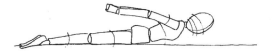

4. Interlace your hands behind your back and raise a little farther yet. Hold a few seconds and collapse (oops! I meant relax).

ABDOMINAL STRENGTHENING

1. **Lie on your back, knees bent, feet flat on floor.**

2 **Place your hands on your prominent front hip bones.**

3. **Flatten lower back against the floor by contracting your abdominal and gluteal muscles and slightly tucking your tailbone under.**

4. **Hold this position (do not let your hip bones move and do not let your lower back lift from the floor) while you alternately pick each foot up off the floor in a "marching" movement.**

   As you pick up one foot, hold it momentarily, then put it down and immediately pick up the other foot. *(Keep breathing relaxed.)*

   For the exercise to be effective, you must keep the tension in the abdominal muscles; do not allow the pelvis to move or the lower back to lift off the floor as you lift your feet.

5. **Repetitions: 5–10 for each leg. You can work up to 25–30 if you like.**

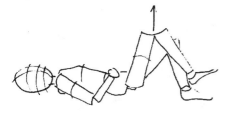

This exercise strengthens your abdominal muscles safely without placing compressive forces on the vertebral column.

CHAPTER V

BALANCE

BALANCE IS A COMPLEX FUNCTION. It depends on visual cues (eyesight), auditory cues (hearing), muscle strength, posture, the sensation of the feet on the ground, and movement and awareness of head position.

Poor balance leads to increased risk of falling and increased risk of a fracture. A fall that results in a hip fracture is life-threatening, especially in the elderly population—a large percentage of those who sustain a fracture do not survive the surgery necessary to fixate the hip; another percentage do not live even a year after the fracture. Of those who do survive, many are limited in mobility and/or are living in an assisted care facility or nursing home. Clearly, prevention is of utmost importance.

DO YOU HAVE A PROBLEM WITH BALANCE?

Can you stand on one leg without holding onto anything? The ability to stand on one leg is closely linked to walking safely and efficiently; when you walk, you stand on one leg as you pick up the other one. If you walk with a halting, shuffling type of gait (which actually increases your risk for a fall), you may be doing so because you are unable to stand on one leg as you pick the other one up.

How fast do you walk? Generally speaking, it is more difficult to walk slowly and maintain balance. So, if you walk fast it may be that you are compensating for a balance problem. Try walking very slowly, picking up each foot very deliberately and maintaining your balance on the other foot—you may be surprised how difficult this is.

When you are moving around your home, do you find yourself touching the walls or furniture just to give yourself that little extra sense of security? This is another indication of a balance problem. Try walking without touching anything and see how you do.

Do you have a fear of falling? Studies show that persons with a fear of falling are more likely to fall.

HERE IS A SIMPLE TEST TO CHECK YOUR BALANCE

Stand in a safe place next to a support you can hold onto if you need to. Try to stand on one leg for 20 seconds, then the other leg for 20 seconds. Hold onto the support as little as possible but as much as necessary. If you cannot do this without holding on, or if you have a great deal of difficulty doing it (or are wobbly), you have a balance problem.

Even if you have no difficulty with balance now, it is a good idea to spend a little time to work on improving and maintaining your balance. Doing so can help prevent falls when you grow older.

The following group of exercises are designed to improve balance. If your balance is poor, do them every day. Stay close to a counter or furniture for support, just in case you need it.

STAND TALL

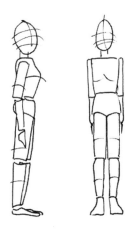

1. **Stand with good body alignment, your feet directly underneath your hips, and with your toes pointed straight ahead.**

   This position may make you feel a little pigeon-toed but it brings your legs and feet into better alignment.

2. **Distribute your body weight evenly between your feet.**

3. **Press your feet into the floor, tighten your knee caps, tighten your buttocks, and tuck your tailbone very slightly.**

4. **Lift your chest and increase the space between your pelvis and your rib cage.**

5. **Lengthen your neck and pretend you are 2" taller** *(see page 13).*

   Do not tilt your head back.

Practice this posture frequently and whenever you are standing for any length of time (in line at the super-market, talking on the phone, etc.).

This exercise (1) helps to strengthen the back; (2) replaces faulty posture with a better one; (3) can help you get out of the habit of always standing on one leg.

BODY SWAY
(2 VERSIONS)

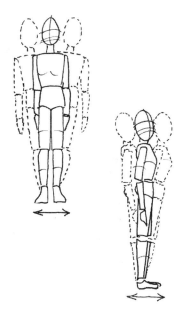

SIDE-TO-SIDE

1. **Stand with your feet directly underneath your hips, toes pointed straight ahead.**

2. **Sway your body from side to side, transferring your body weight from one leg to the other. Move only at your ankle joints.**

   Keep your body straight. It should move as if it is a solid structure all the way from your ankles to the top of your head. Do not pick up your feet, do not bend your knees, do not bend at the waist.

3. **Repetitions: 5–10.**

FORWARD–BACKWARD

1. **Stand with your feet directly underneath your hips, toes pointed straight ahead.**

2. **Sway your body forward and backward, onto the balls of your feet and then back onto your heels.**

   Once again, the movement occurs only at your ankles and your body should move as if it is a solid structure. This movement is very small. Do not pick up your heels or your toes as you sway.

3. **Repetitions: 5–10.**

These two exercises help to strengthen your legs and to evenly distribute your weight between your two legs.

ONE-LEG STANDING

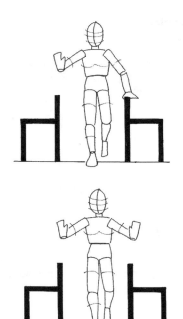

1. **Stand with good body alignment, feet directly underneath hips, with toes pointed straight ahead. Support your hands on each side.**

   You can use 2 chairs, a kitchen counter and a chair, etc. Whatever you use should be at your sides so that you do not have to bend forward for support.

2. **Transfer your weight onto your right leg; pick up your left foot.**

   You are standing on your right leg.

3. **If you are steady, pick up your right hand.**

   You are now supported by your right leg and left hand.

4. **If you are steady, pick up your left hand.**

   You are standing on your right leg with no other support.

5. **Stand on your right leg for up to 20 seconds, with good body alignment.**

   The exercise will not be as effective if you are wobbling from side to side to maintain your balance. (For help in remaining steady, focus your eyes on an object at eye level.)

6. **Lower your hands and left foot, so you are again supported by both feet and both hands.**

7. **Transfer weight onto your left leg, pick up your right foot, your left hand, and then your right hand.**

8. **Repetitions: 1–2 times for each side.**

When you can stand on each leg for 15–20 seconds, you will have good one-leg balance, and you will notice improvement in your overall balance and ability to walk steadily.

COORDINATED WALKING

1. **Stand with a counter or railing at your side, with your feet directly underneath your hips and toes pointed straight ahead.**

2. **Walk FORWARD along the counter.**

   Use walking techniques on pages 59–60.

3. **Walk BACKWARD along the counter.**

   The toe is the first part of the foot to come down on the floor.

4. **Turn and face the counter, toes and knees facing forward, and hold on lightly if you need to.**

5. **Step SIDEWAYS with your left leg, then bring your right leg over to meet it. Continue to step and close sideways for as long as you have room.**

6. **Reverse direction.**

7. **Repetitions: 3–5.**

This exercise will (1) strengthen your legs, back and hip muscles; (2) improve your overall balance and your balance while walking.

DYNAMIC WEIGHT SHIFTING

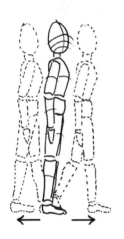

1. **Stand with your feet directly underneath your hips and with your toes pointed straight ahead. Support your hands on each side.**

   If needed, hold onto a support (such as the kitchen counter or 2 chairs); hold on as much as you need to but as little as possible and still be safe.

2. **With your left foot in place, STEP FORWARD ONTO YOUR RIGHT FOOT, transferring your weight onto the right leg. Hold for a moment, then transfer your weight BACK ONTO THE LEFT FOOT. Now step BACK WITH YOUR RIGHT FOOT and place your weight on it.**

3. **Shift weight back and forth by moving the right leg forward and backward 6–10 times.**

4. **Repeat sequence, standing on the right leg and moving the left leg forward and backward 6–10 times.**

This exercise benefits the leg that you are standing <u>on</u> because it teaches you to transfer your weight through the hip joint as you move the opposite leg forward and backward. In this way, you are exercising the muscles around the hip of the standing leg, strengthening them and allowing the weight of your body to go through the entire range of the hip.

CHAPTER IV

WALKING

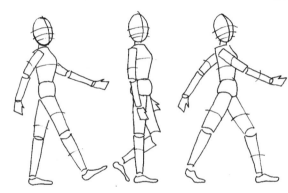

Misalignment of the hip may contribute to osteoporosis of the hip and osteo- arthritis of the hip and knee, as well as to low back pain.

WALKING IS THE SINGLE BEST all-around exercise that can be done by the most people at nearly any time. Whenever I announce that I am going to teach a class on walking, one of the responses I frequently get is, "Why do I need to take a class to learn how to walk? I've been walking for 30 or 40 (or 70 or 80) years. I think I know how to walk."

My answer is that, although you have been walking for several decades, you may not be getting all you can out of it because of poor body alignment or poor gait mechanics.

Walking, a weightbearing exercise, helps combat osteoporosis because body weight passes through the hip joint—that is, if you walk properly. If you are like most people, however, you probably have tightness in certain muscle groups in the hip area causing a forward tilt of the pelvis. When you walk (actually, when you stand on one leg, which is part of walking), the weight passes in front of the hip joint instead of through it. This misalignment of the hip may contribute to osteoporosis of the hip, osteoarthritis of the hip and knee, as well as to low back pain.

HOW TO WALK

- Follow the visualizations in Chapter I as you walk. Pretend that:
  ...a plumb line has been dropped beside your body—stay "in plumb."
  ...you are 2 inches taller than you are.
  ...a rope attached to the top of your head is pulling you up.
  ...a hook attached to your breastbone is pulling you upward.
  ...someone has hold of the scruff of your neck and is pulling you up.

- Pull yourself up in an effort to lengthen the space between your rib cage and your pelvis (waist area).

- Lengthen your spine.

- Practice the "bucket": keep your pelvis level by contracting your buttocks and abdominal muscles; gently tuck your tailbone under or, if you are already tilted backwards, stick your tailbone out slightly.

- Heel/toe: touch the heel of each foot to the ground first (the toes leave the ground last).

- Arm swing: feel the natural swing of your arms in opposition to the movement of your legs (a natural movement that helps to balance the body as your walk), then exaggerate the swing.

- Long legs: imagine that your legs actually start at the back of your waist; use your large buttock and upper thigh muscles to "push-off" and give animation to your walk.

- Pull/push: pretend that someone is pulling you along by a rope attached to your belly button, or is pushing you along with their hands on your buttocks.

- Feet-like-feathers: walk lightly—pretend that each foot is a feather as it touches the ground.

- Straight line: walk in a straight line; try to eliminate any side-to-side movement of your body.

- Breathe evenly as you walk.

At this point you are probably saying, "wait a minute . . . there is no way that I can remember all of that at the same time."

And you are right.

You won't remember all of it at the same time. So just remember one thing and concentrate on it. Then go on to the next thing. Before you know it, you will put it all together and be walking with improved body alignment and energy, and you will be strengthening your body at the same time.

HOW TO GET THE MOST OUT OF YOUR WALKING

• Keep a regular schedule, and walk for at least one-half hour, 4 times a week. If you are unable to walk this long at a time, and your tolerance is only 5 minutes, then start with 5 minutes, and gradually build in time and intensity. Walking time should be uninterrupted.

• Exercise for your heart: when you walk, you are also exercising your heart. To gauge the intensity of your walking and its effect on your heart, you may want to get a heart rate monitor and follow a conditioning program (*see* "Heart Zone Training" from The Heart Zone Training Assn., 2636 Fulton Ave., Sacramento, CA 95821; phone 1-800-959-4089.)

• Wear good, supportive shoes. Your shoes act as a shock absorber for your body; they help eliminate the shock forces that are transmitted up through the knees, hips, and lower back. You should invest in a good pair of walking shoes.

In general, get shoes that are long enough with the toe box wide enough to give your feet plenty of room to spread out while bearing your weight. Most people wear shoes that are too short and/or too narrow, which results in foot pain and deformity such as bunions, hallux valgus and hammer toes.

When you buy shoes, shop late in the day when your feet may be slightly swollen; if the shoes fit then, they will fit at other times as well. Don't buy too-narrow shoes thinking that they will give and conform to your feet. Your feet will give out long before the shoes, and you will likely discard both the shoes and your walking program.

As a rough guide as to whether a shoe is too narrow, hold the bottom of the right shoe against the bottom of your left foot (and vice versa). The shoe must be wider than your foot because your feet spread a little when you stand on them.

• Walker/Cane: If you use an assistive device such as a walker or a cane, continue to do so as you begin your walking program. As you improve in strength and stability, you may be able to graduate from walker to cane to no device at all.

DON'T FORGET TO HAVE FUN!!!

Smile and have fun while you walk. Walk with a friend. Walk in an interesting place—just be sure you are safe.

You will be surprised at all the parts of the world you have missed while riding around in a car. You will see flowers and trees. The neighborhood will look different. You can have a whole new outlook on life just by adding walking to your daily routine. And . . . you will be strengthening your bones to boot!

CHAPTER IV

SCAPULAR STABILIZATION

THE FOLLOWING FIVE EXERCISES strengthen the muscles between your shoulder blades. These muscles are important for body alignment and good posture and help to stabilize the shoulder girdle for safe movement of the shoulder joints. Another benefit of these exercises is that they help increase your shoulder range-of-motion.

You will be using a resistive band (such as a Thera-Band®), which provides resistance to movement. Although the exercises can be done seated or standing, it is better to start by lying on your back. In this position, your back is supported and stable so that you can move your arms without twisting your body and without injuring your shoulders.

GENERAL INSTRUCTIONS

Lie on your back with your knees bent (feet flat on the floor), feet pointing straight ahead, feet and knees hip distance apart. If you have been able to do the other exercises with legs extended and knees straight, and have had no strain or discomfort in your back, you can do the same for these exercises, although for isolation of shoulder movement it is better to have knees bent.

Start each exercise with 5 repetitions. If that is too many, then start with 3. Work up to no more than 10 repetitions for each exercise.

Breathe out as you do the movement of each exercise.

Do not hold your breath.

After you have mastered the exercises, you may want to increase the resistance with a different band; the bands are color-coded so you can tell which resistance you are using.

THE OVERHEAD

1. **Lie on your back as in the Decompression Exercise** *(page 20)*.

2. **Grasp the band with both hands at about hip level, elbows straight and palms down.**

3. **Pull the band outward to the sides, then bring arms up and back overhead as far as you can.**

   Keep elbows straight and keep tension on the band throughout the movement. (*Breathe out as you move your arms overhead.*)

4. **Hold position 2–3 seconds, then bring arms down to hip level.**

5. **Repetitions: 3–10.**

This exercise is easier with the hands far apart and harder with the hands closer together.

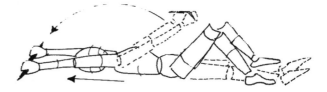

THE SIDE PULL

1. **Lie on your back as in the Decompression Exercise** *(page 20)*.

2. **Grasp the band with both hands at about hip level, elbows straight and palms down.**

3. **With elbows straight, bring arms up to a right angle with the body.**

4. **Keeping elbows straight, pull the band out to the sides.**

   Your hands will come down to the floor and the band will cross your collarbone. (*Breathe out as you move your arms out to the sides.*)

5. **Hold 2–3 seconds, then return to the starting position (#3).**

6. **Repetitions: 3–10**

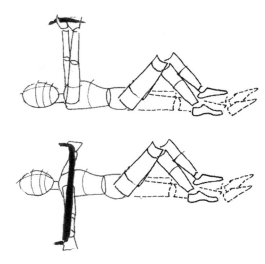

THE SASH

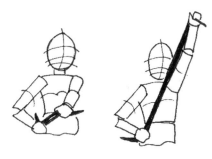

1. Lie on your back as in the Decompression Exercise *(page 20)*.

2. Grasp the band with the right hand, and place it on your right prominent front hip bone.

3. With elbow straight and thumb pointed downward, bring left hand up in the air over your navel.

4. Starting with some tension on the band, pull the left arm up diagonally and overhead, so the band crosses your chest like a sash.

   Keep elbow of the moving arm straight throughout the movement. Tension on the band will increase as you pull on it. (*Breathe out as you move your arm diagonally and overhead.*)

5. Hold 2–3 seconds, and return to the starting position (#3).

6. Repetitions: 3–10.

7. Change sides and repeat with right arm 3–10 times.

ARM ROTATION

1. Lie on your back as in the Decompression Exercise *(page 20)*.

2. Grasp the band with your hands turned toward your face. Bend elbows to a right angle and tightly tuck them into your sides.

3. Pull band apart, bringing hands down toward the floor.

   If you are unable to pull your hands apart with your elbows tucked and bent, move one arm at a time, then try both together.
   (Breathe out as you move your arms outward.)

4. Hold position 2–3 seconds, then return to the starting position.

5. Repetitions: 3–10

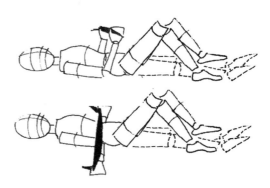

BOW AND ARROW

1. Lie on your back as in the Decompression Exercise *(page 20)*.

2. Grasp the band with both hands; bring arms straight up in front of you until they are at a right angle to your body, and your hands are about 5–7 inches apart.

3. With your left elbow straight, pull right arm down, bending the elbow at the same time (as if to shoot an arrow from a bow).

   (Breathe out as you move your arm downward.)

4. Hold position 2–3 seconds, then return to the starting position (#2).

5. Repeat the movement 3–10 times with right arm.

6. Repeat #3, #4 and #5, keeping the right elbow straight and pulling down with the left arm.

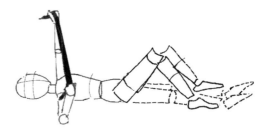

CHAPTER VI

ACTIVITIES OF DAILY LIVING

A regular exercise program will be more effective if it is accompanied by the practice of good body mechanics during regular daily activities.

THESE ARE THE THINGS you do every day of your life: brushing your teeth, getting in and out of bed, cooking a meal, walking the dog.

If you have osteoporosis, it is vital that your routine activities are conducted with good body mechanics, which will help prevent compression fractures, reduce your risk of a fall, and alleviate back pain. If you do not have osteoporosis, good body mechanics are important for the prevention of back pain and injury.

As you consider each activity, observe where you are making mistakes and begin changing your habits. This is not easy, I know. But it will be worth it. Your reward will be less back pain, prevention of back injury, and increased function in everything you do.

Two instructions apply to many activities:

1. Don't bend at the waist—bend your knees and kneel or squat;

2. Don't reach unnecessarily—get close to the activity. But when you must reach, a "golfer's reach" is easier on your back *(see picture on page 79)*.

Some conditions—knee pain or poor balance, for example—may make it hard or even impossible to practice good body mechanics. In that case, the use of the following assistive devices is helpful:

1. A reacher: an all-purpose, long-handled gadget that has pinchers, a hook, and usually a magnet at its far end. This device assists in reaching items without effort.

2. A long-handled shoehorn and elastic shoelaces (so you can put on and take off your shoes without untying them).

3. A long-handled bathbrush, so you can reach without twisting or bending.

STANDING

To improve your body alignment (posture), press your hips forward over your knees and under your shoulders.

If you have to stand for a long time—which can place stress on the lower back, causing pain—place one foot on a low stool, alternating feet. Wear flat shoes and maintain good body alignment.

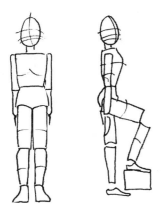

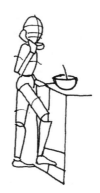

TALKING ON THE TELEPHONE

Whether sitting or standing, take time to find a position with good body mechanics.

Do not lean the phone on your shoulder; either hold it or get a phone support that allows your hands to be free without leaning your head to the side.

If your job requires a lot of talking on the phone, ask your employer to furnish you with head phones.

Do not run to answer the phone.

STAIRS

Stay close to the railing and use it as needed. Wear shoes that give stable support, avoid those (such as high heels and "scuffie" slippers) that do not. Avoid restrictive clothing or long flowing robes that can get caught on the steps or trip you if you step on them.

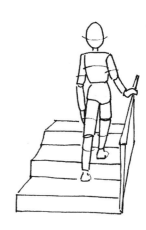

SITTING

Sitting—especially sitting with a forward lean—is the position of greatest compression on your back and is not a position of choice. Most people do far too much sitting.

Sit upright and support your lower back with a rolled-up towel or lumbar support in the hollow area of your lower back. Relax your shoulders. Do not slouch and do not cross your knees for very long.

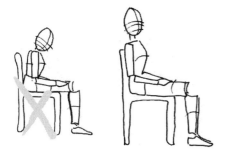

SITTING AT THE COMPUTER: Support your lower back as above. Make sure your head is not tilted upwards as it will be if you wear reading glasses and look through the lower part. You may need a special pair of "computer glasses" that are focused at monitor-distance. Do not lean forward

READING: Sit upright; rest reading material on a pillow or a tilted support. When seated in a recliner or easy chair, support your elbows on the arm rests; this will help support your back. Change position frequently. Get up to stretch at least once each hour.

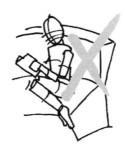

EATING: Follow rules for sitting. Do not lean over the table or rest head on hands. Bring your food to your mouth, not your mouth to the food.

SITTING DOWN (from standing)

Bend your knees as you lower your body onto the chair; "stick out your tailbone" toward the back of the chair. Use your hands for support and sit down gently; do not "plop" into the chair. Imagine you are going to sit on an egg and don't want to crack the shell.

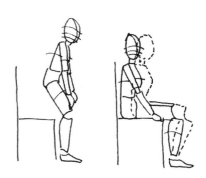

STANDING UP (from sitting)

Move to the front of the chair. Place one foot slightly in front of the other; bend at the hips (like a jackknife); keep your back straight as you stand up. Use your hands, keep your chest up, and avoid "giving way" at the waist.

LIFTING, PUSHING, PULLING, CARRYING

The rules for lifting are the same, no matter how light the item is. Body position is what matters.

- Stay close to the item.
- Keep your feet shoulder width (or further) apart or place one foot in front of the other.
- Always bend your knees (kneel or squat), to avoid strain on the back.
- Bend your knees when reaching (or use a reacher).
- Pushing is better than pulling.
- Keep object as light as possible (remove part of contents, if you can). If item is heavy, get help.
- Do not twist or bend your back. Turn by moving your feet, not pivoting and twisting on one leg.

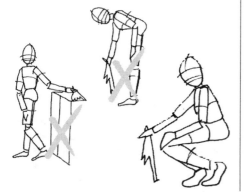

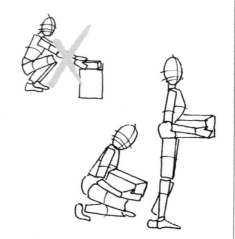

TO LIFT FROM THE FLOOR

Slide the item up onto one thigh. Use both hands to hold it close to you at waist level, then stand up.

TO LIFT AND MOVE

Stay close to the item. Keep your back in good alignment, and let your leg muscles do the work.

TO MOVE FURNITURE

Do it very carefully, following the rules for lifting (at left). When lifting with another person, both lift at the same time. If you have osteoporosis, do not move heavy furniture by yourself.

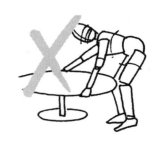

PUSHING VS. PULLING

Pushing is better than pulling. Keep your back in good alignment, and let your leg muscles do the work. Keep your elbows at your sides and use total body weight and leg strength.

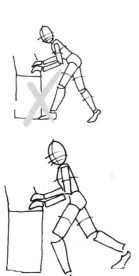

PUSHING A WHEELCHAIR

Stay close to the chair; do not bend your back or lean forward. Bend your elbows and keep arms close to your sides; use your legs and push with your whole body.

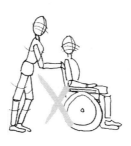

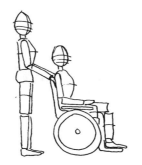

CARRYING A SUITCASE

Use wheeled luggage or a cart. If you must carry a suitcase, use your body as one unit, with weight distributed evenly on both sides. Do not twist your trunk.

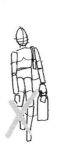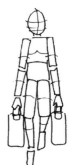

CARRYING A POCKETBOOK

Keep it light—check contents periodically and take out unnecessary items.

If you use a shoulder bag, alternate shoulders or place the strap across your chest.

If you use a fanny pack, wear it in the back; it helps keep your arms free and improves body mechanics. (In questionably safe areas, wear it in the front.)

IN THE BEDROOM

GETTING INTO/OUT OF BED

These are the safest ways, with the least compression on your back.

SIDEWAYS METHOD: Sit on edge of the bed.

Lower your body down onto one side. Support yourself on your arms as you bend your knees and bring legs and feet up onto the bed.

Now roll over on your back.

To get up, reverse movements.

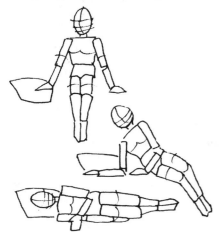

HANDS AND KNEES METHOD: On the bed, get onto your hands and knees. Lower your body down onto one hip, then onto your side.

Now roll over onto your back.

To get out of bed, use the sideways method.

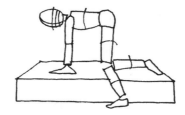

SITTING UP IN BED

Do NOT sit straight up in bed. This movement causes too much stress on the vertebrae and could cause a fracture. Instead, use the sideways method, pictured at left.

TURNING OVER IN BED

Always move your body as one unit.

If you are lying on your back, bend your left knee, place your left arm across your chest, and roll to the right.

Bend your right knee and keep your knees together when on your side.

Reverse movements to turn the other way.

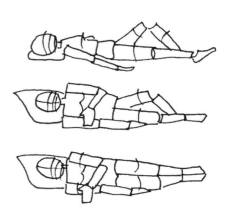

LYING IN BED

LYING ON YOUR BACK: This is your best sleeping position, as it is the position of least compression for your back. For added comfort, place small pillows under your knees and neck, and possibly a towel roll under your waist.

Lie in this position several times a day, especially when your back aches *(see The Decompression Exercise, page 20).* As a preventive measure, lie on your back *BEFORE* your back starts to ache. You will have more success at relieving the pain than if you wait until you are in severe pain.

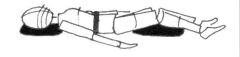

LYING ON YOUR SIDE: Don't curl up into fetal position because it causes too much bending of the spine and hips, and contributes to postural problems and spinal compression.

To reduce strain on your lower back, place a pillow between your knees to prevent the upper leg from falling forward onto the bed. Use a support under your neck and around your waist. A pillow wedged behind or under you and perhaps a pillow in front will help you maintain good body alignment.

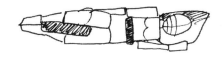

LYING ON YOUR ABDOMEN: Place a pillow under your lower legs and under your stomach, chest, and/or hips as needed. Rest head on chin or forehead or on hands with hands turned palms down or turn head to the side supported with a small pillow.

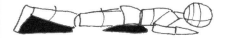

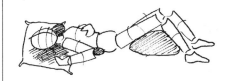

SEXUAL INTERCOURSE

When you have osteoporosis, sexual intercourse is potentially dangerous unless you are careful about positioning. Avoid forward bending movements as much as possible.

You should be aware that both you and your partner are living with the problem. Start by agreeing to put a special effort into your relationship; bring the sensuality and understanding as well as the sexuality back in.

For more information regarding this area of your life, I recommend the book *Sex and Back Pain* by Lauren Hebert, P.T. (IMPACC USA, publisher, 1 Washington St., Greenville, ME 04441).

IN THE BATHROOM

USING THE SINK

When brushing your teeth or washing your face, do not bend your back—bend your knees instead.

Open the cabinet and place one foot up on the shelf.

For putting on make-up or shaving, use a mirror on a stand that you can bring closer to you instead of leaning toward the mirror over the sink.

USING THE TOILET

Follow rules for correct sitting *(page 71)*. Bend your knees as much as possible as you sit down. You may need to install grab bars for hand support (the sink, toilet paper holder and towel rack are NOT good supports).

Place the toilet paper where you can reach it without twisting.

If you have trouble getting up and down, consider installing an elevated toilet seat.

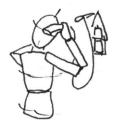

TAKING A SHOWER

Standing in the shower is safer than getting into the tub for a bath. If standing is a problem, get a shower chair. Consider using a hand-held shower and/or a long-handled back brush. Use a non-skid mat in the tub *and* on the floor outside of the tub.

GETTING DRESSED

Never dress while standing on one leg, especially if you have balance problems. Sit to put on pants, then stand to pull them up.

Sit on the toilet or edge of the bed to put on your shoes and socks. Bring your foot up instead of reaching down to your feet.

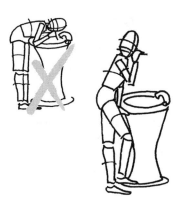

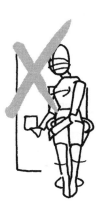

IN THE KITCHEN

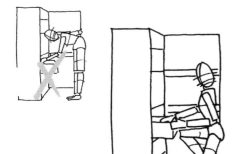

COUNTER WORK—WASH, CHOP, MIX, COOK

For standing, the ideal countertop height is no lower than 2-4" below elbow level; seated, it is at elbow level. To wash dishes in the sink—especially if you are tall—raise the tub by placing it on a turned-over pot.

Stand close to your work. Limit reaching and avoid bending forward at your neck or waist. Open a lower cupboard door and place one foot on the shelf.

LOAD/UNLOAD DISHWASHER

Kneel, squat, or sit in a chair. Place items to load, or just unloaded on the counter so you don't have to bend, twist, or reach. Consider using just the top shelf.

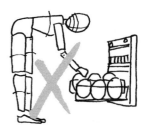

REFRIGERATOR

Keep frequently used and heavier items on an easy-to-reach shelf (waist level). Have the door open so you can place items from the refrigerator onto a counter next to it; if your refrigerator opens the other way, the hinges can be changed.

Bend your knees or squat down to reach the crisper; do not bend your back. Or store vegetables and fruits in plastic bags and use a reacher to put them into/out of the crisper.

When you buy a new refrigerator, consider one with a bottom freezer.

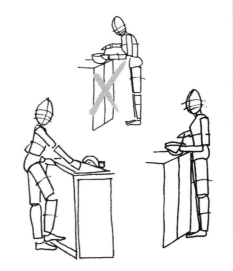

77

HOUSEWORK

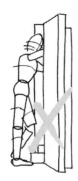

Set up good work conditions. Remove clutter from closet floors, for example, so you can get closer to the shelves. You will also be less likely to trip.

MAKING THE BED

Squat down; don't bend your back. Walk around the bed; don't reach.

If your bed is against the wall, place one hand and one knee on the bed to reach pillows or straighten covers, or use a reacher. Use lightweight bedding, such as a down comforter, and extra-depth fitted sheets.

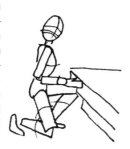

GETTING ITEMS FROM A LOW SHELF

Don't bend over; squat down or kneel instead. Raise one leg out behind you ("golfer's reach") as you reach down into a cabinet. Use a lazy susan to keep items within reach. Use a reacher.

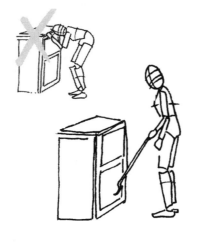

GETTING ITEMS FROM A HIGH SHELF

Shift your weight from your front foot to the back foot as the item is lifted off the shelf. Don't stand on tip-toes; use a sturdy stool, preferably one that locks as you stand on it or one that has a handle for support.

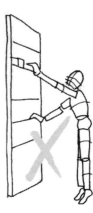

LOADING/UNLOADING THE WASHER

To load, place the basket where you won't have to bend and twist.

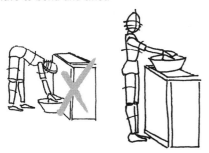

To unload items from the bottom, reach into the washer with one arm and lift the opposite leg behind you (golfer's reach). Or use a reacher.

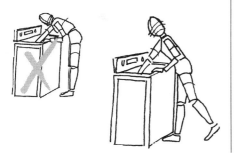

LOADING/UNLOADING THE DRYER

For a front-loading dryer, place items on the open door. If the door does not form a shelf, kneel or squat, use a stool as a shelf, or use a reacher. Do not bend your back. Place small items in a zippered bag.

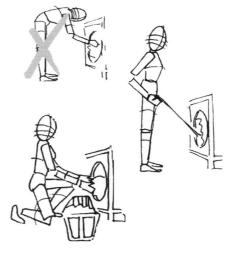

Consider buying a stackable washer/ dryer combination.

IRONING

Proper height of the ironing board is very important; it should be high enough so you do not have to lean forward as you iron. When ironing for a long time, put one foot on a small stool to relax your back.

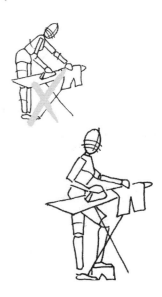

HOUSEWORK

DUSTING/CLEANING

Stay as close to your work as possible. To reach farther away, kneel or squat, and use your knees instead of your back. Use a long-handled duster or window-washing sponge. Be careful climbing ladders and never stand on the top step.

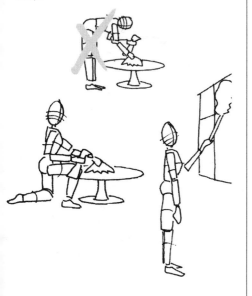

SWEEPING

Hold the broom close to you. Don't reach or twist; walk over to the dirt. Use a long-handled dustpan and don't bend over.

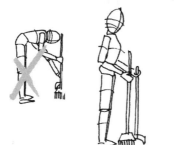
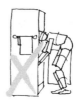

VACUUMING

Hold the vacuum close to you at hip level. Don't reach or twist; step back and forth with the vacuum.

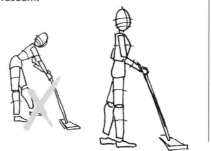

CLEANING THE TUB

Kneel on one or both knees or squat down; don't bend your back. Reach the corners with a long-handled sponge or brush.

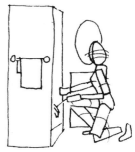

BABY CARE

PICKING UP BABY FROM FLOOR

Squat or kneel down and bring the baby close before picking him/her up. Use your knees, not your back. Do not pick up a child who is old enough to climb into your lap.

TWO-STAGED LIFT: Lift baby onto a chair or sofa first; then stand and complete the lift.

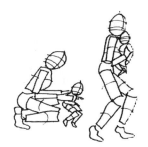

FEEDING THE BABY

Use pillows to help position both you and the baby so that both of you are comfortable and your back is supported.

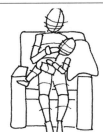

PUTTING BABY INTO A CARSEAT

Get as close as you can to the task; if you can, place one foot inside the car. Bend your knees to avoid back strain. Avoid twisting movements. Let child climb in if he/she is old enough.

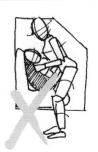

GIVING BABY A BATH

To lift baby into or out of the tub, squat down or kneel close to the edge of the tub. Use a non-skid mat in the tub and a non-skid rug on the floor. Use a seat for the baby if he/she is old enough to sit—then your hands are free to bathe and play with the baby. Never leave a baby unattended, even for a moment.

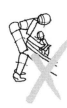
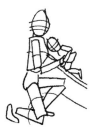

IN AND OUT OF CRIB

Have child stand if possible. Be sure to lower the side rail.

DIAPER CHANGE

Make sure the surface is high enough to avoid bending your back.

YARDWORK

RAKING

Place upper hand under the handle. Stay close to the work area. Keep your back straight and stable and use arm movements to do the work. Do not reach or twist.

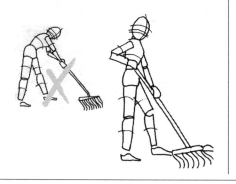

SHOVELING (dirt or snow)

Push from the end of the handle and shift body weight back and forth so that you are using as much body weight as possible to help. Keep your knees slightly bent and avoid twisting your back.

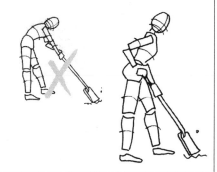

PULLING A CART

Pull the cart alongside of you while walking. Don't bend your back or twist. When reaching into the cart, lift opposite leg and keep your back straight. A self-balancing cart is better and safer than one that tilts.

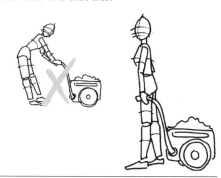

PLANTING AND WEEDING

Squat or kneel down instead of bending your back. Use knee pads or a kneeling pad with handles. Consider a wheeled stool. Use lightweight, long-handled tools that are designed for easy handling .

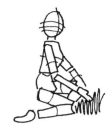

DIGGING

Dig small amounts of earth at a time. Insert the shovel as vertically as possible and use body weight to push into the earth.

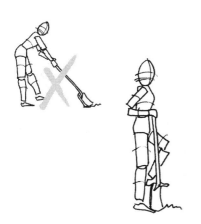

MOWING

Keep up with the mower as you are moving along. Avoid reaching and letting the mower get too far in front of you.

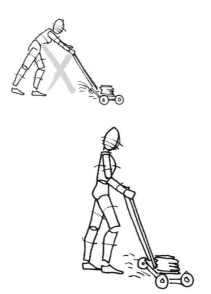

PET CARE

When picking up a small dog or cat, keep your pet close to you and follow the rules for safe lifting.

Use a reacher to pick up empty bowls

When walking the dog, keep the leash at your side—DO NOT let the dog pull you along. Consider using a retractable leash.

For grooming, place your pet on a table where you can more easily reach. Otherwise, kneel or squat down to the floor.

To lift your pet into or out of a tub, squat down or kneel close to the edge of the tub. Bathe small animals in a sink.

THE CAR

GETTING IN/OUT OF THE CAR

Lower your body onto the seat. Move back on seat, then bring one leg into the car at a time. If sliding on the seat is difficult, place a plastic bag on the seat.

Reverse movements to get out of the car.

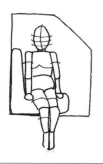 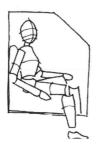

DRIVING

Before driving, adjust the seat and steering (if you have tilt control) to ensure good posture. Use a towel roll or lumbar support behind your back. Fasten seat belt.

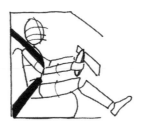

SHOPPING

When reaching into the shopping cart with one hand, lift the opposite leg behind you (golfer's reach). Stabilize yourself by holding onto the cart.

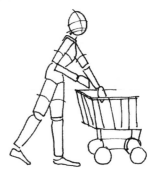

GETTING ITEMS FROM TRUNK

Try to maintain the curve of your lower back when reaching into a deep trunk.

Use one hand for support.

Reach into the trunk with the other hand and raise the opposite leg behind you (golfer's reach).

Have groceries packed in small bags.

Ask for help with large items.

Slide items close to you before lifting.

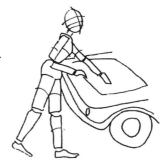

CHAPTER VIII

WHAT'S NEXT?

AFTER YOU HAVE COMPLETED the exercises and activities in this book, you may be wondering where you can go from here. Because this program begins at a very low level, building in difficulty and intensity, it paves the way for you to take the next step, which may be to a fitness center, gym, exercise class, or to some specific sport.

By now, you have learned principles of exercise and movement that will help prevent injury. But you still need to be cautious in many environments and class situations.

IF YOU HAVE OSTEOPOROSIS OR OSTEOPENIA

If your bones are fragile, the exercises and movements you *shouldn't* do are just as important as those you *should* do. Use extreme caution when following an exercise program on television, videotape, or in a class in a senior center— such programs frequently contain movements and exercises that you definitely should not do.

Here are some guidelines:

Avoid any exercise where there is forward-bending (flexion) of the trunk over the legs or bringing the knees toward the chest. They can cause increased compression on the vertebral column and could result in compression fractures. What to avoid: abdominal crunches, sit-ups, straight leg raises, knee-to-chest exercises, toe touches (either from a seated or standing position), and any exercise where you simultaneously bend and twist the trunk.

Although you have gained much strength in your back extensor musculature and have improved your posture, your bones are still weak and you may place yourself at risk for a vertebral fracture. (Also, because most postural problems are the result of too much forward movement, these types of exercises are not necessary.)

Pool exercise

Exercising in the water is fun, stimulating, and makes you feel good all over. It is more or less weightbearing depending upon the depth of the water; movement through the water places resistance forces on the bones. As always, avoid forward bending or flexion movements.

Walking in the pool (water walking) is excellent for strengthening the legs and improving range of joint motion. Follow the same guidelines as walking on land (see pages 59–62).

Swimming is also good exercise as it increases flexibility and endurance. Be sure to include the back stroke, breast stroke, and side stroke to offset the postural problems (tight, forward shoulders) that can result from the freestyle.

Yoga

Yoga is an excellent form of exercise but you should approach it with caution. Though back alignment is emphasized, there are many forward-bending postures that should be avoided or done in perfect alignment under supervision of a skilled teacher in order to eliminate compression of the vertebral bodies. Tell your yoga teacher about your condition and ask him/her to watch your movement and to critique you, to make certain you are keeping your back stable and straight. Substitute extension exercises for the flexion ones.

T'ai chi

T'ai chi is very popular and has been shown to improve balance. The movements are slow and controlled and should pose no risk. Avoid any forward-bending of the back. Look for a qualified teacher, preferably one who has been trained by a T'ai chi master.

Seated exercises

Exercising in the sitting position can be very stressful on your back because sitting is the position of most compression on your back. If you exercise in the seated position, support your lower back with a rolled-up towel or special back support, and keep your back straight and stable by lifting your chest. Avoid forward-bending movements.

Aerobic exercise

Aerobics are good for your cardiovascular system, but you should avoid high impact aerobics. Walking and low impact aerobic exercise will give you plenty of cardiovascular conditioning. Follow the visualizations and suggestions for body alignment when doing aerobic exercise.

Tennis, golf, bowling

These sports should be approached with great caution. Because they include bending and twisting type movements and because they are very "one-sided," they pose a great risk for back injury. If you have osteoporosis, I suggest that you consult a physical therapist who can review your body mechanics and can make suggestions for your increased safety.

Going to the gym or fitness center

A certain amount of caution is needed. Personal and one-on-one training are very popular. Unfortunately, your personal trainer may not be aware of the risks associated with osteoporosis. Again, avoid any forward-bending exercises or any machines that strengthen the muscles that pull you forward (such as the PecDeck or bench press). With any exercise, be sure your back is stabilized and supported. Avoid stationary bicycles and spinning classes. Freeweights are far superior to machines.

IF YOU DO NOT HAVE OSTEOPOROSIS OR OSTEOPENIA

With normal bone density, you may add some forward-bending movements to your program. If you do not know your bone density, you should get a bone density test to find out.

A good fitness program includes a balance of flexion, extension, and rotary movements. Most people find forward bending easier to do and so avoid extension (backward-bending) movements; but unless you have a balance of these two movements, you could end up with more postural problems and back pain.

In summary, a regular physical exercise program will help you in your quest for better health. No matter what age you are now, what you do *NOW* can help you achieve a more independent old age.

GLOSSARY

ABDOMINALS – group of muscles located on the front of the body between the ribs and pelvis; their action is to bend and twist the body forward and to help support the back and abdominal cavity.

ASSISTIVE DEVICE – term physical therapists use to describe such items as walkers, canes, quad canes, crutches, reachers, long-handled tools.

BACK (REGIONS OF) – low back: from the top of the pelvis to the rib cage; mid-back: from the lower rib cage to area between the shoulder blades; upper back: from level of the shoulder blades to the nape of the neck.

COMPRESSION – refers to pressure on the vertebral bodies. Too much compression can cause a compression fracture, which is a collapse of the vertebral body, usually in a forward direction.

DECOMPRESSION – in osteoporosis, there is excess compression on the vertebral bodies. The exercises in this program are designed to decompress the vertebrae.

EXTENSION – backward movement of the body. In an extension exercise, the body is moved backward from the neutral position (or back to neutral, if the body is too far forward).

EXTENSORS (BACK) – the deep layer of muscles of the back; also called the erector spinae, paraspinals, back strap muscles, and anti-gravity muscles. These important muscles hold your body up against the force of gravity. Neglected in most exercise programs.

FLEXION – forward bending of the body. In a flexion exercise, the body is bent forward or the knees are brought toward the chest. Contraindicated in people with osteoporosis because of the risk of a compression fracture.

GLUTEALS – large group of muscles located in the buttocks area; they are weak and under-used in people with postural problems and forward flexed posture.

HAMSTRINGS – group of muscles located on the back of the thigh; their action is to extend (straighten) the hip and bend the knee.

LUMBAR LORDOSIS – the curve of the low back between the rib cage and the pelvis. An exaggerated lumbar lordosis is sometimes called swayback.

LUMBAR SPINE – lumbar area of the spine; same as the low back.

LUMBAR SUPPORT – a support for the low back (lumbar) area; can be purchased at a medical supply or drug store, or fabricated from a rolled-up towel or small pillow.

OSTEOPENIA – precursor to osteoporosis; a weakening of the bony structure; diagnosis is by bone density scan.

OSTEOPOROSIS – condition in which the bones are deficient in minerals to the extent that fractures occur easily; diagnosis is by bone density scan.

REACHER – assistive device for picking up objects from floor, pulling out low drawers, etc. Eliminates the need to bend the back and/or knees when reaching.

ROTATOR CUFF – group of four muscles located deep in the shoulder joint, which maintain the integrity of the shoulder joint. May be injured from a quick movement with a position and/or weight that cannot be supported by the shoulder.

SCAPULAR DEPRESSION – movement of the shoulder blade downward.

SCOLIOSIS – an abnormal side curve of the vertebral column.

SHOULDER GIRDLE – the area of the shoulder joints, shoulder blades, and collar bones.

SITE-SPECIFIC EXERCISE – an exercise designed to affect the bone to which the exercised muscle is attached; also, to stretch and strengthen specific areas of the body to restore good body alignment.

THORACIC KYPHOSIS – curve of the vertebral column from the nape of the neck to just above the waist. An exaggeration of this curve is often called a dowager's hump.

TOWEL ROLL – a support for your lower back or neck you can make by rolling up a towel.

INDEX

Names of exercises
appear in italics

(def.) = defined in glossary

A

Abdomen, protruding, 10
Abdominal muscles, 89 *(def.)*
    exercises for, 35, 36, 51, 49
Abdominal Strengthening, 51
Aerobic exercise, 87
    walking, 61
Alternate Hip Extension, 43
Angels in the Snow, 34
Ankle Pumps/Calf Stretch, 27
Ankle, exercises for, 23–24, 26
Arm, exercises for, 30, 37, 41, 63–68
Arm Lengthener, 30
Arm Press, 33
Arm Rotation, 67
Assistive device, 62, 69, 89 *(def.)*

B

Baby care, 81
Back
    alignment, exercises for, 20, 22, 28, 29,
      31, 37, 47, 49
    extensors, 10, 89 *(def.)*
    flexibility, exercises for, 37
    lower, exercises for, 23–24, 26
    lying on, 16, 18, 75
      tolerance for, exercise, 20
    pain, 9, 10, 11, 12, 15, 17, 19, 59, 69, 88
    regions of, 89 *(def.)*
    relaxing, 18

Back, continued
    exercises for, 21, 29, 31, 35, 36, 42, 43,
      44, 45, 46, 48, 50
    strain, 16, 17
Balance, 11,17, 52–53
    exercises, 54–58
    test, 53
Bathtub, how to clean, 80
Bed
    back safety in, 74–75
    making, 78
Belly Press, 42
Bench press, 88
Body mechanics, 12, 69–84, 87
Body Sway, 55
Bone density and exercise, 15
Bone density test, 9
Bow and Arrow, 68
Bowling, 87
Breathing, 18, 19, 60, 63
Bridging, 35–36
Buttocks, *see* Hip muscles
Buttock Squeeze, 25

C

Calf muscles, exercises for, 23–24, 26, 27
Cane, 62
Car, getting into/out of, 84
Cat (The), 37
Carrying, 72–73

Chest muscles, exercises for, 21, 28, 29, 31, 34, 38, 39, 40, 44–46, 49
Chin Tuck/Head Slide/Head Press, 22
Cleaning the house, 80
Combination Exercise, 50
Compression (spinal), 11, 15, 18, 19, 71, 89 *(def.)*
   exercises to relieve, 18, 20, 21, 29, 31, 49
   fractures, 15, 69, 86
Computer, sitting at, 71
Coordinated Walking, 57
Cover the Bones, 31

D

Decompression, 89 *(def.)*
Decompression Exercise (The), 18–19, 20
Digging, 83
Disc problems, 11, 15, 19
Dishwasher, using, 77
Dowager's hump, *see* Thoracic kyphosis
Dressing, 76
Driving, 84
Dusting, 80
Dynamic Weight Shifting, 58

E

Elbow Press, 28
Exercise(s), 10, 11–12, 15, 16
   aerobic, 87
   balance, 11, 52-58

Exercise(s), continued
   breathing and, 18, 19
   bucket, 14
   decompression, 18–19, 20
   frequency, 15
   length of session, 16
   muscle soreness and, 17
   order of, 16
   pool, 86
   repetitions, 16
   scapular stabilization, 11–12, 64–68
   site specific, 11, 15; *see also* Spine, exercises for
   osteoporosis and, 9, 85, 88
   seated, 87
   visualization, 11, 13–14, 59–60
   walking, 11, 59–62
   weightbearing, 11, 59, 86
Extension, 15, 89 *(def.)*
Extension-in-Standing, 40
Extensors, back, 10, 85, 89 *(def.)*
   exercises for, *see* Back, exercises for
Extensors (hip), *see* Hip muscles

F

Falling,11, 52, 53, 69
Fitness center, 88
Flexion, 37, 85, 86, 88, 89 (def.)
Forward-bending, *see* Flexion

Fracture risk, 9, 10, 52, 85

G

Gardening, 82
Gluteals, 89 *(def.)*
Golf, 87
Golfer's reach, 69

H

Hamstrings, 42, 43, 48, 89 *(def.); see also* Hip muscles
Head
   exercise to align, 22
   exercise to hold up, 22, 47
Head Lift, 47
Heel cords, exercises for, 23, 24, 41
Heel Extender, 24
Hip Extension (Alternate), 43
Hip fracture, see Fracture risk
Hip muscles, exercises for, 23–24, 25, 26, 35, 36, 40, 42, 43, 48, 49
Hip joint, weightbearing through, 59
Housework, 78–80

I J

Improvement, lack of, 18
Injury, old, 17
Ironing, 79
Jewel, showing off, 14

K

Knee position for exercises, 17
Knee muscles (back of), exercises for, 26
Knee-to-chest, 10, 85
Kyphosis, *see* Thoracic kyphosis

L

Leg Lengthener, 23
    Variations, 24
Leg Press, 26
Leg exercises, *see* Calf; Heel cord; Knee
Leg Straightener, 24
Leg/Arm Lift, 48
Lifting, 72
Low back, 17*; see also* Back pain
Lumbar lordosis, 17, 90 *(def.)*
Lumbar spine, 90 *(def.)*
Lumbar support, 90 *(def.)*
Lying in bed, 75
Lying on back, as exercise, 18

M N

Making the bed, 78
Mental Imagery, *see* Visualization exercises
Morning Stretches, 32
Moving furniture, 72
Mowing lawn, 83
Muscle soreness, 17
Neck structures, exercises for, 22, 47

O

One-Leg Standing, 56
Osteoarthritis, 59
Osteopenia, 19, 85, 88, 90 *(def.)*
Osteoporosis, 9-10, 11–12, 15, 19, 59, 85, 88, 90 *(def.)*
Overhead (The), 64

P

Pain, 12, 13, 18; *see also* Back pain
Pelvis, level, 14
Pet care, 83
Plumb line, 13–14, 59
Pool exercises, 86
Posture/correction, 11–13, 15, 63, 86
Pulling, 72–73, 82
Pushaways, 41

R

Pushing, 72–73
Raking leaves, 82
Range of motion, 18, 30
Reacher, 69, 90 *(def.)*
Reaching, 78, 84
Rotator cuff, 90 *(def.)*
Rounded shoulders, exercises for, 21, 28, 29, 31, 34, 38, 39, 40, 41, 44, 45, 46, 49, 50, 63–68

S

Sash (The), 66
Scapular depression, 90 *(def.)*
Scapular stabilization, 11–12, 63
    exercises for, 64–68
Scoliosis, 90 *(def.)*
Sexual intercourse, 75
Shoes, for walking, 61–62
Shoulder Blade Squeeze, 44–46
Shoulder girdle, 90 *(def.)*
Shoulder Press, 21
Shoulder Retraction, 38
    with Depression, 39
Shoulders, exercises for, 21, 28, 29, 30, 31, 32, 33, 34, 38, 39, 41, 44, 45, 46, 48, 63–68
Shoveling, 82
Showering, 76
Side pull (The), 65
Sink, using, 76
Sit-ups, 10, 85
Site-specific exercise, 11, 15–19, 90 *(def.)*
    for the spine, *see* Spine
Sitting, 71, 74, 87
Slipped disc, 11, 15, 19, 90 *(def.)*
Sphinx (The), 49
Spinal compression, 11, 15, 18, 19, 71
    exercises to relieve, 18, 20, 21, 29, 31, 49
    fractures, 15, 69, 86

Spine, exercises for, 20, 21, 22, 25, 26, 28, 29, 31, 35, 36, 37, 42, 43, 44, 45, 46, 47, 48, 49, 50
Spondylolisthesis, 11, 15, 19
Stairs, 70
Stand Tall, 54
Standing, 70, 71
Straight leg raises, 10, 85
Suitcase, carrying, 73
Sweeping, 80
Swimming, 86

T

T'ai chi, 87
Telephone, talking on, 70
Tennis, 87
Thera-Band, 63

Thoracic kyphosis, 90 (def.)
    exercises to lessen, 13–14, 20, 21, 28, 29, 31, 44–46, 49
Thoracic Lift, 29
"Tie high," 14
Think taller, 13
Toe touches, 10, 85
Toilet, using, 76
Towel roll, 90 *(def.)*
Turning over in bed, 74

V

Vacuuming, 80
Vertebral bodies, *see* Spinal Compression
Visualization exercises, 11, 13–14, 59–60

W

Walker, 62
Walking, 11, 59-61
    balance and, 52—53
    Coordinated, 57
    shoes for, 61–62
    in the pool, 86
Washer/dryer use, 79
Weeding, 82
Weightbearing exercise, 11, 59, 86
    through hip joint, 59
Wheelchair, pushing, 73

Y

Yardwork, 82—83
Yoga, 86

Order Form

Please send me

____ copies WALK TALL (spiral binding) @ $16.95 per copy + shipping/handling *(see table)*.

____ TheraBand® resistance bands* (yellow) @ $1.50 (ordered & shipped with book)

____ TheraBand® resistance bands* (yellow) @ $6 (ordered alone; shipping included)

Ship to: Name _____

Address (street address) _____

City/State/Zip _____ Phone _____

Add 6% sales tax for items sent to Florida addresses.

To charge to your credit card:

☐ Visa   ☐ MasterCard   ☐ Discover   ☐ American Express

Cardholder's name _____

Card number _____ Expiration date _____

Mail to: Triad Publishing Company
P.O. Box 13355, Gainesville, FL 32604
With credit card: fax order to 1-800-854-4947

SHIPPING & HANDLING CHARGES, PER ADDRESS

	CONTINENTAL US	ALASKA, HAWAII, US TERR.	CANADA
Up to $30	$6	$8	$15
$30 to $80	$8	$12	$20
$80 to $200	$10	$18	$25

Shipments to cont. U.S. and Canada are sent by UPS surface; to Alaska, Hawaii, U.S. territories by airmail. Foreign orders, inquire (specify air or surface); charges payable in U.S. funds drawn on a U.S. bank, or by credit card. Fax queries to 325-373-1488.

Thera-Bands® are color-coded with graded resistance; tan is the lowest resistance, followed by yellow, red, green, blue, black, silver, and gold. They are available from physical therapists and medical supply stores.

RELATED BOOKS AND ITEMS

I would like to receive information about:

☐ STAND TALL! EVERY WOMAN'S GUIDE TO PREVENTING AND TREATING OSTEOPOROSIS, by Morris Notelovitz, M.D. Current facts about osteoporosis; what can be done to prevent and/or treat it.

☐ SAVE YOUR BONES! HIGH CALCIUM, LOW CALORIE RECIPES FOR THE FAMILY, by Lois Goulder. 96 pages, 73 recipes plus meal planning and shopping suggestions.

☐ NOT JUST CHEESECAKE! A YOGURT CHEESE COOKBOOK, by Shelley Melvin. 250 delicious recipes, from appetizers to desserts, featuring yogurt cheese. Quick, easy preparation.

(OVER)

☐ MIKE'S FAMOUS YOGURT CHEESE MAKER. Easiest way to make high-calcium, non-fat yogurt cheese; delicious replacement for cream cheese, sour cream, and whipped cream. And it's fun!

☐ Sara Meeks' videos for everyone:

( ) OSTEOPOROSIS, PATIENT EDUCATION. Designed to answer questions about osteoporosis.

( ) BODY ALIGNMENT, BALANCE, GAIT MECHANICS. With the help of Patty, a woman with osteoporosis, Sara presents her program for improving posture, improving balance, lengthening and strengthening the back, and walking with emphasis on weightbearing through the hip joints.

☐ Sara Meeks' videos for physical therapists:

( ) BACK STABILIZATION AND POSITIONING

( ) SPECIFIC STRETCHING OF THE HIP AND KNEE

( ) BALANCE AND RESISTANCE BAND EXERCISES